Metabolic Magic

The Short Course To A Super Slim Physique

BY ROBERT KENNEDY
& DWAYNE HINES II

Copyright 2000 By Robert Kennedy

All rights reserved including the right to reproduce
this book or portions thereof in any form whatsoever.

Published by MuscleMag International
5775 McLaughlin Road
Mississauga, ON Canada
L5R 3P7

Designed by Jackie Kydyk
Edited by Matt Lamperd

Canadian Cataloguing in Publication Data

Kennedy, Robert, 1938-
　　Metabolic magic: the short course to a super slim physique

ISBN 1-55210-023-5

　　1.Reducing exercises. 2. Reducing diets. I.Hines, Dwayne, 1961- II.Title.

RA781.6.K45 2000　　646.7'5　　C00-901322-9

Distributed in Canada by
CANBOOK Distribution Services
1220 Nicholson Road
Newmarket, ON
L3Y 7V1
(800) 399-6858

Distributed in the States by
BookWorld Services
1933 Whitfield Park Loop
Sarasota, FL 34243

Printed in Canada

Warning
This book is not intended as medical advice, nor is it offered for use in the diagnosis of any health condition or as a substitute for medical treatment and/or counsel. Its purpose is to explore advanced topics on sports nutrition and exercise. All data are for information only. Use of any of the programs within this book is at the sole risk and choice of the reader.

Table of Contents

Chapter One
Getting On Track 5
Chapter Two
Weight Lifting For Weight Loss 9
Chapter Three
Fighting Fat: Cutting Carbs 15
Chapter Four
Fiber For Fat 21
Chapter Five
Long and Moderate Cardio/aerobic Workouts 27
Chapter Six
The Metabolic Program 33
Chapter Seven
20 Tips & Techniques To Hype Your Metabolism 37
Appendix A
Calorie Chart For Burning Off Bodyfat 46
Appendix B
Eating Right 46

CHAPTER ONE

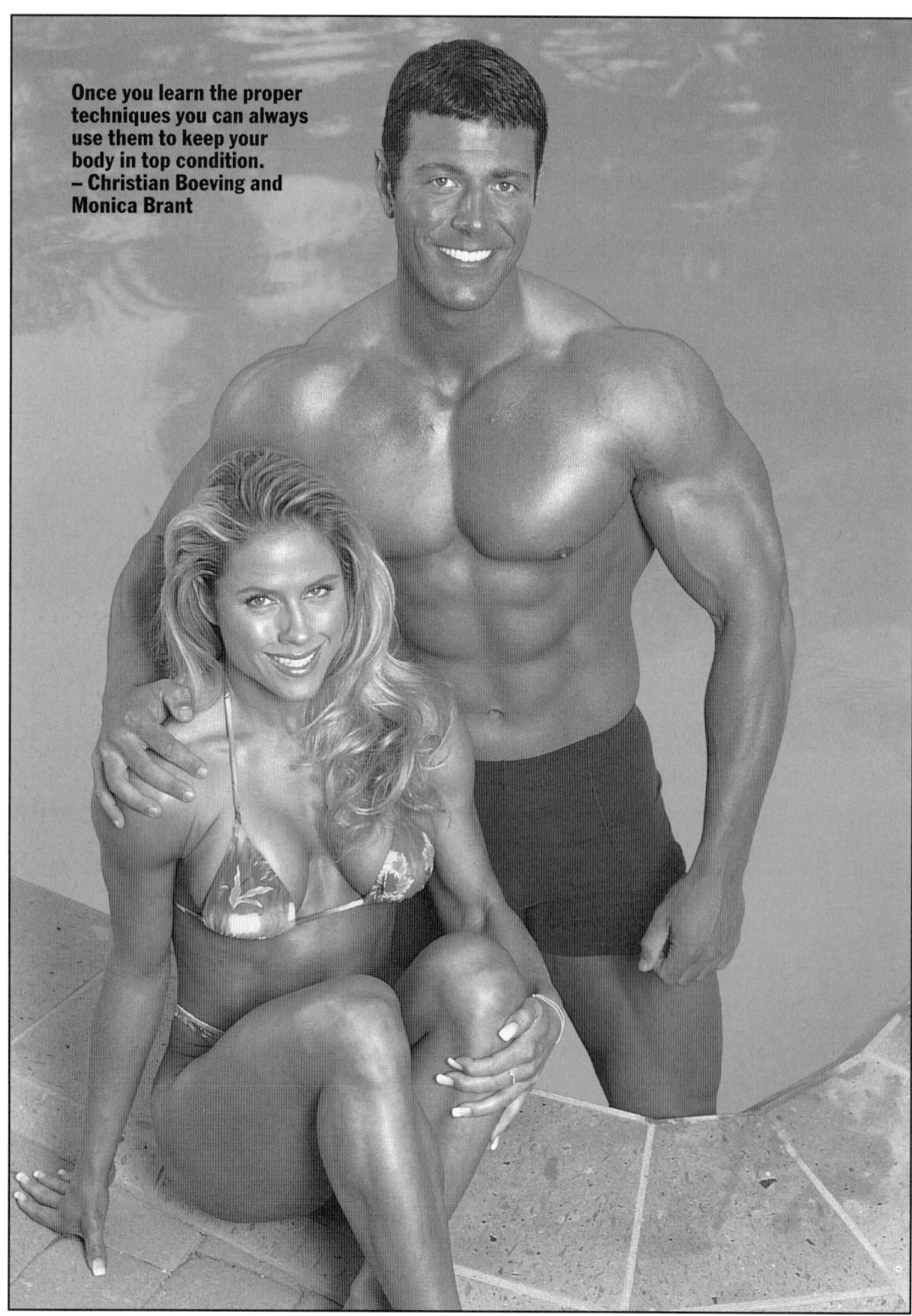

Once you learn the proper techniques you can always use them to keep your body in top condition.
– Christian Boeving and Monica Brant

Getting on Track

Would you like a shapely, yet trimmer physique? A better question might be "who wouldn't?" Someone once said that you can never be too rich or too thin. Yet obtaining a slim physique for many people seems to be about as easy as becoming a multimillionaire. It has been noted that about 90 percent of the people who go on a diet eventually gain back all the weight they lost plus more within a couple of years. Trimming down is even tougher when you have to sort through all of the marketing hype and confusing programs to find something that really works. It almost makes you want to give up before you try anything. Unfortunately, many people do. But that is not the way things have to end up for you. *Metabolic Magic* contains solid, clear, and concise advise, provided in just four simple steps. By understanding and applying these four steps you can get the upper hand on your physique and shape a slimmer body. You don't need some little plastic device that is the latest fad to hit the market (which will disappear shortly thereafter). The information necessary for making significant changes in your physique is not faddish, but based on solid training and dietary techniques. The information in this book can be used year after year as the various fads come and go.

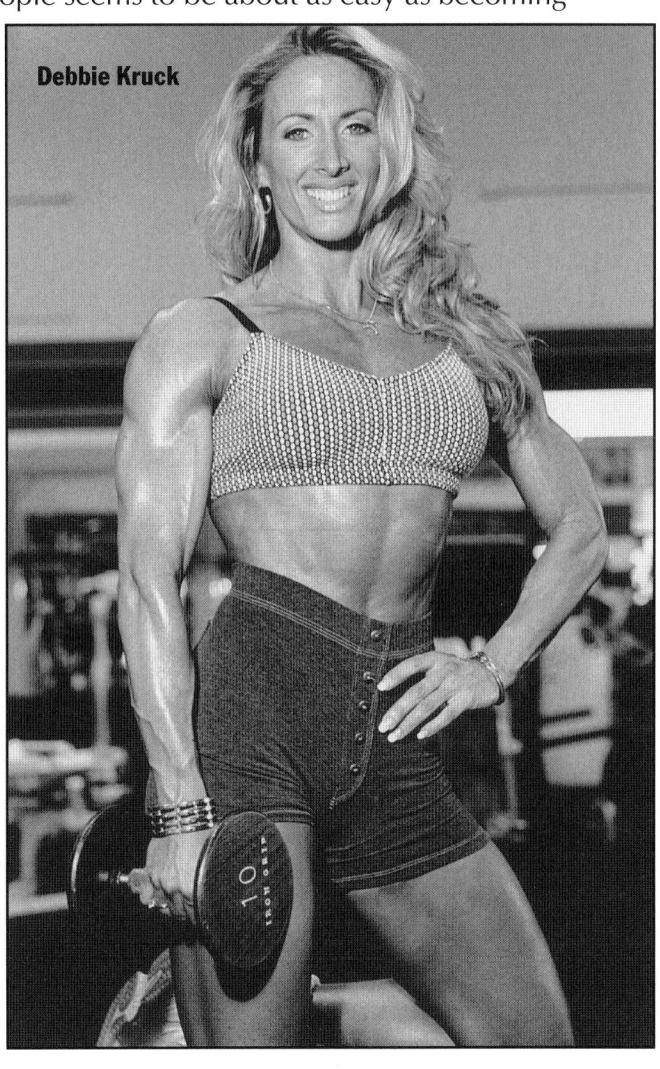

Debbie Kruck

Fads don't last, but solid fitness techniques do. Once you learn the proper techniques you can always use them to keep your body in the desired condition – trim and shapely.

CHAPTER ONE

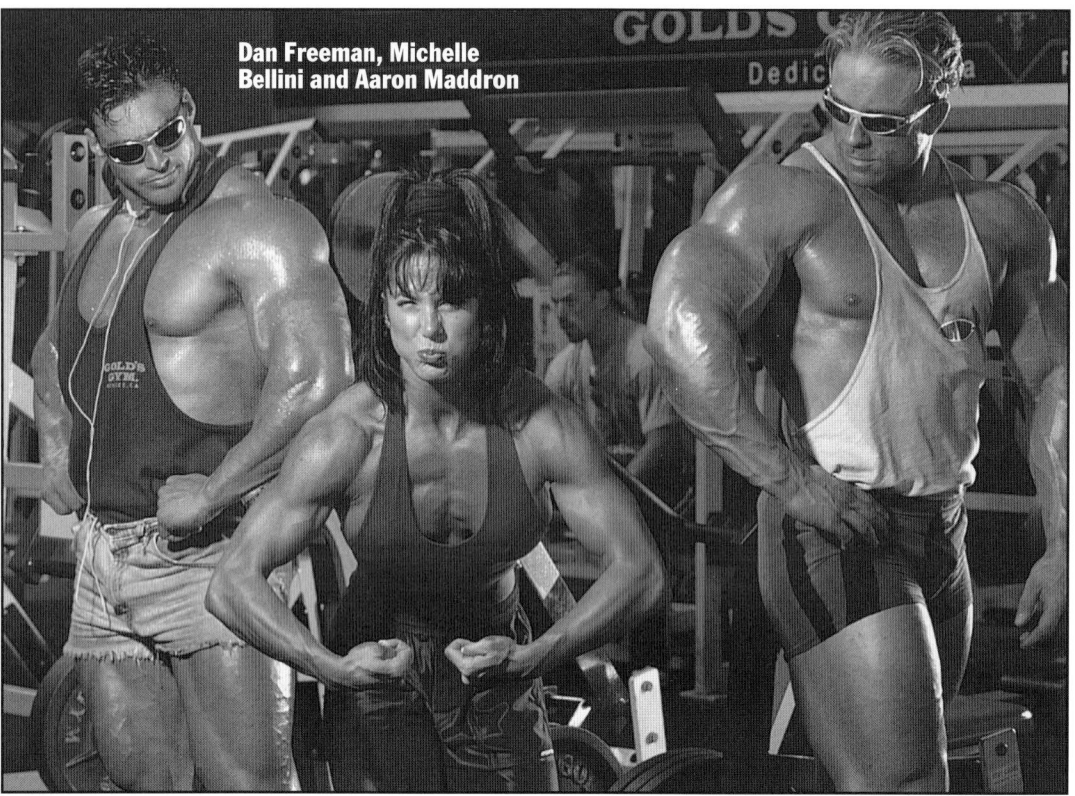

Dan Freeman, Michelle Bellini and Aaron Maddron

Metabolic Magic does not contain complex and confusing information. Sometimes people make fitness more difficult than it needs to be. Acheiving a lean condition is not necessarily easy, (if it was, everybody would be walking around with six-pack abs!); however, it can be done if you are willing to follow the right principles. This book presents the basic body-trimming elements that will enable you to shape a leaner physique.

Consistency

The steps required to slim your physique are presented in this book. All you have to do is apply them in a consistent fashion – make them a habit. If you continuously apply the four elements in this book they will work in your favor, enabling you to shape a super slim physique. Consistency is one of the most important habits you can develop when it comes to working with your body. Hit-and-miss workouts provide a hit-and-miss physique.

You don't have to be rich or famous to shape an awesome physique. Anyone can build a great-looking body. The four slimming techniques are not hard to grasp, but not everyone knows what they are or how to apply them. By reading *Metabolic Magic* you will be well-equipped on what to do and how to do it. *Metabolic Magic* also provides you with the reasoning behind the four trimming techniques.

Metabolic Magic

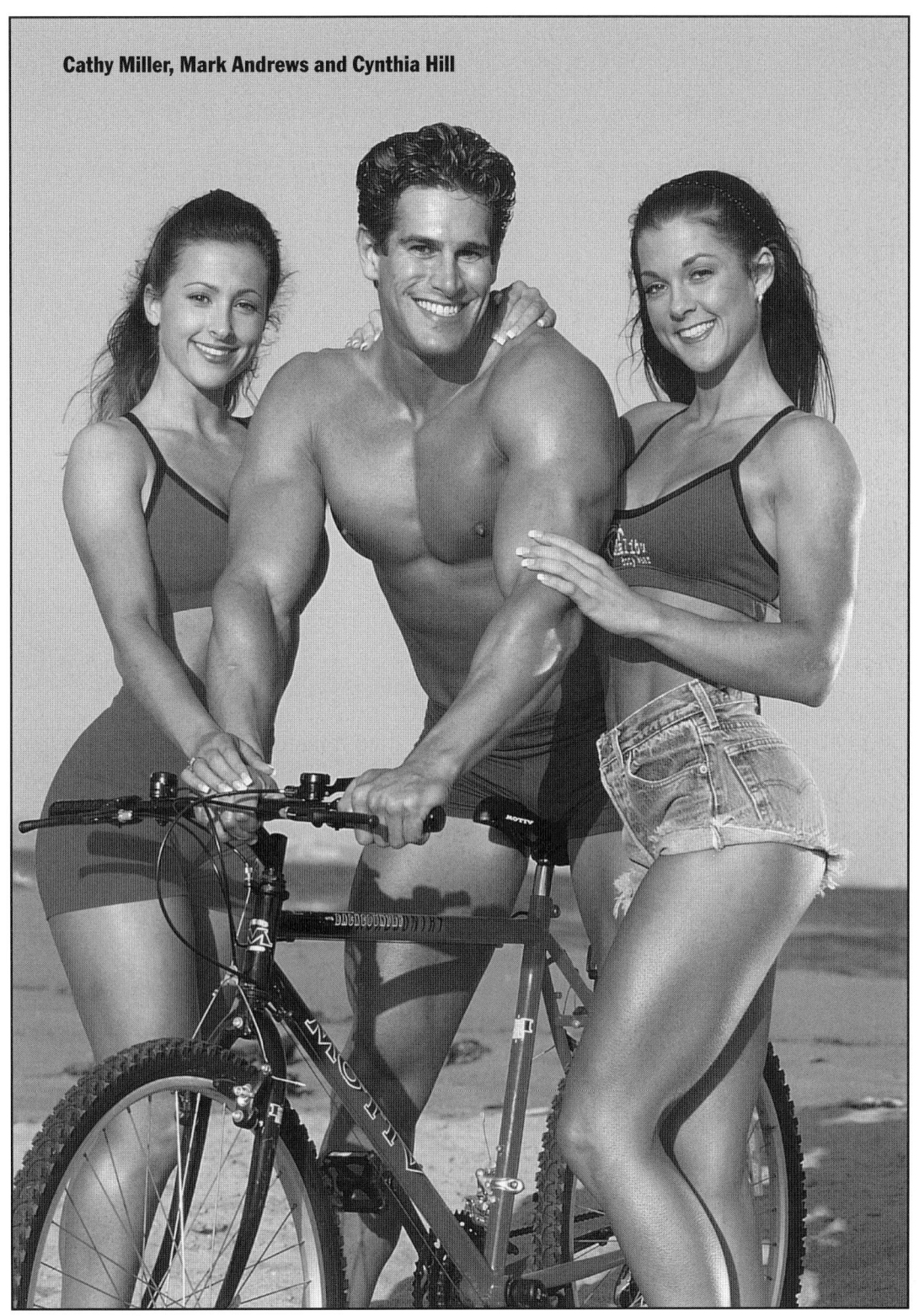

Cathy Miller, Mark Andrews and Cynthia Hill

CHAPTER TWO

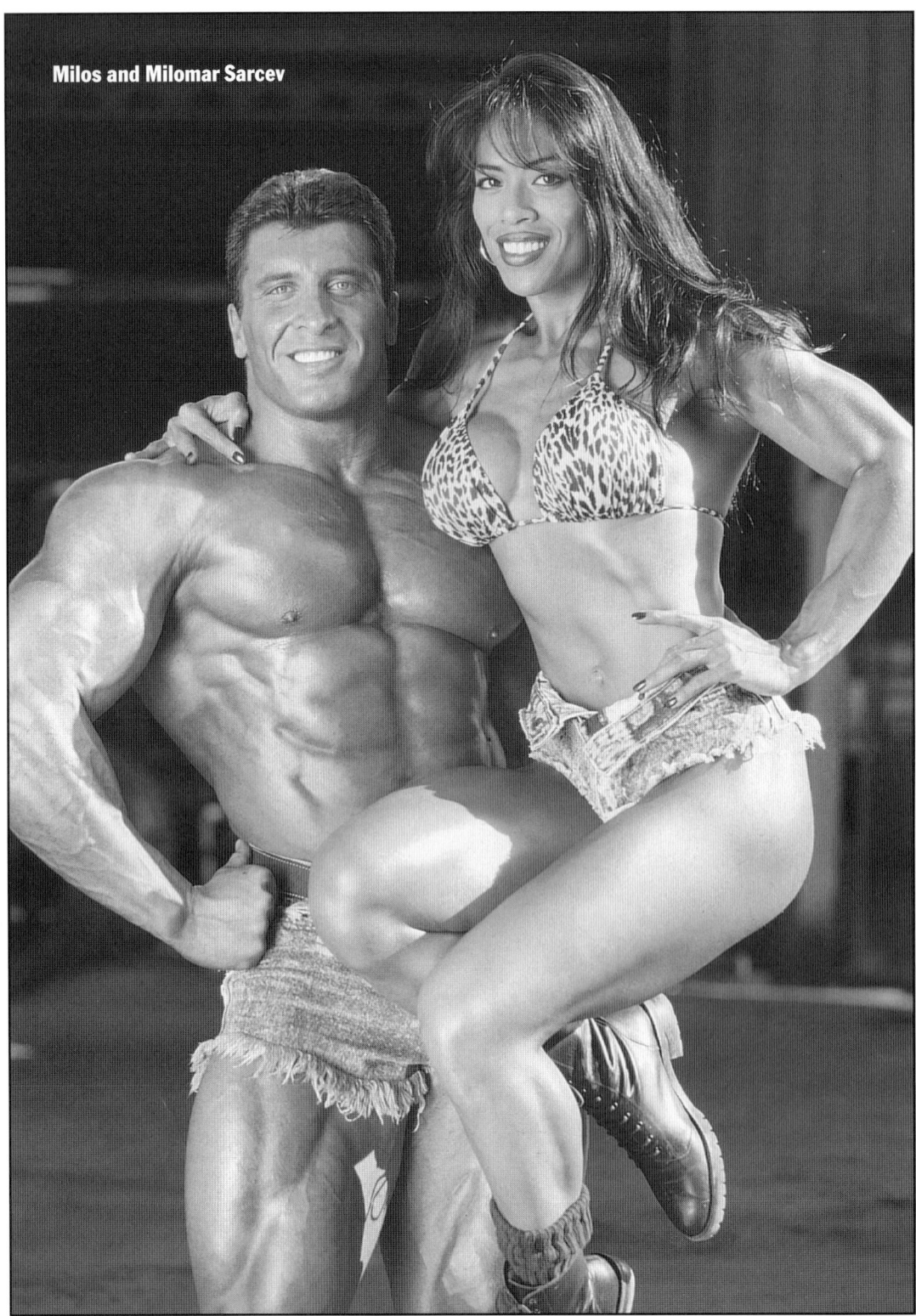
Milos and Milomar Sarcev

Weight Lifting for Weight Loss

Who would have thought that weightlifting and weight loss go together? Most people envision weight gain and big monstrous muscles when weight training is mentioned. It is true that weight training can be used to increase muscle mass, but it also acts to burn off bodyfat.

Fuel Source

Exercise is important for decreasing bodyfat stores. It enhances insulin effectiveness while promoting fat loss and lean-tissue maintenance.[1] When exercise is used to burn off unwanted bodyfat, emphasis is often placed on the fuel source that is used during exercise. Your body uses two primary of fuel during a workout – fat and glycogen. The manner in which the fuel sources are used varies.

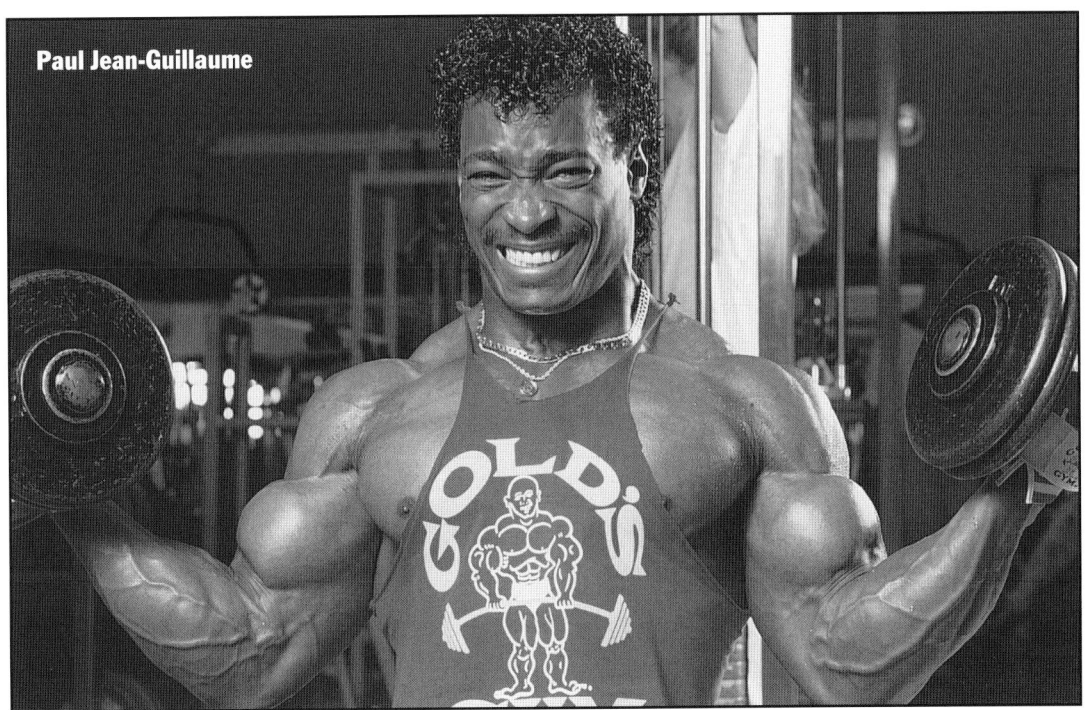
Paul Jean-Guillaume

CHAPTER TWO

Low-intensity exercise tends to burn more fat as a percentage of fuel than does high-intensity exercise. Weight training is a high-intensity exercise. And what does that mean? It means that during a weightlifting workout the body is more likely to use glycogen instead of fat for fuel. But there is another important consideration, the postworkout effect.

The Postworkout Effect

The postworkout effect is even more important to the fat-loss equation than the type of fuel source used during a workout. This element is a crucial factor in the area of fat loss. The postworkout effect centers on what happens after, not during, the workout. And in the postworkout-effect environment, weightlifting is king.

Weightlifting causes your metabolism to rise substantially for a long period after the workout is over. Cardio/aerobic style exercise (such as jogging, biking, etc.) primarily uses fat as a fuel source during the workout (particularly if the workout lasts for over 20 minutes) but weight training primarily uses fat for fuel after the workout. The effect upon the metabolism from cardio/aerobic exercise continues

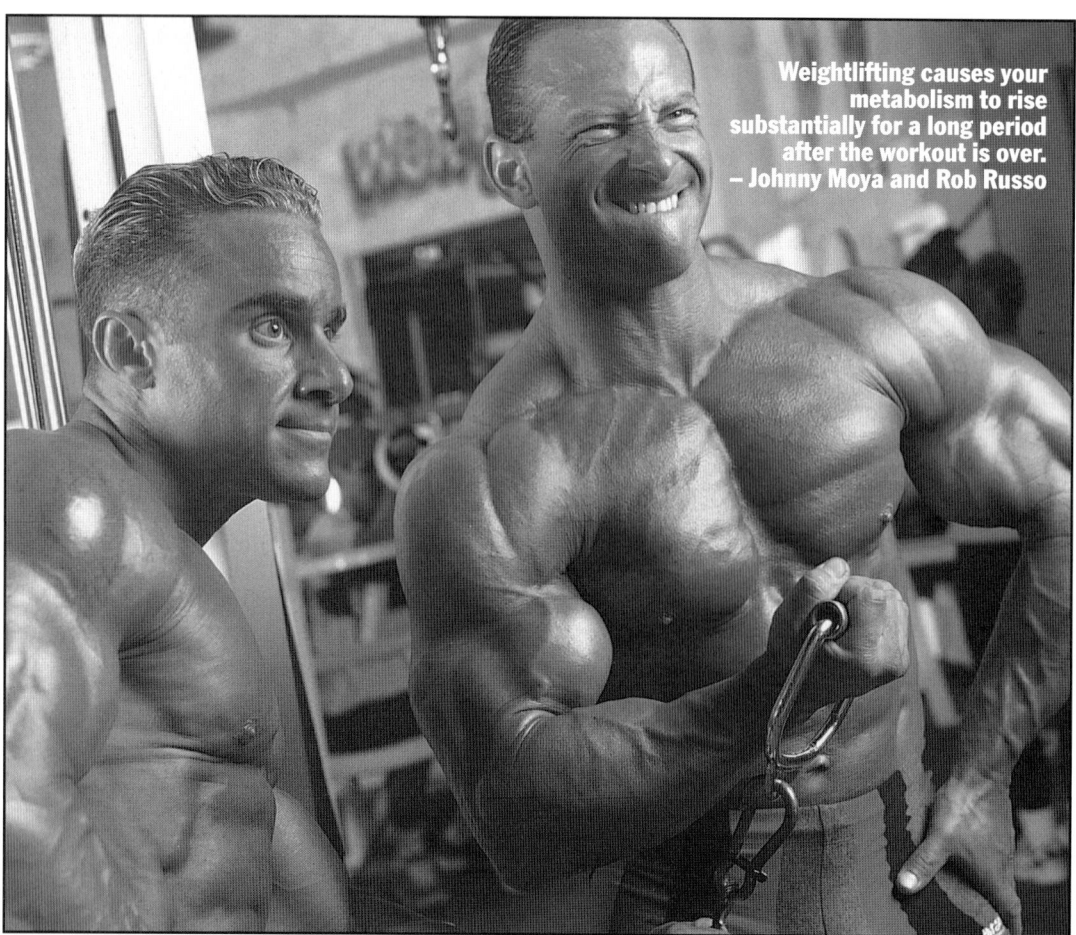

Weightlifting causes your metabolism to rise substantially for a long period after the workout is over.
– Johnny Moya and Rob Russo

Metabolic Magic

for a while and then abates, but the effect of weight training continues long after the workout has ended. An elevated metabolism equates to an increase in fat loss. Since the metabolism plays such a crucial role in burning off bodyfat, "hyping" the metabolism through weightlifting is essential.

Second Favorable Factor

There is a second factor that works in your favor to burn off bodyfat. When you weightlift on a consistent basis you increase your muscularity, which changes your body composition to one of more muscle and less fat. This "shift" greatly aids you in your quest to eradicate unsightly bodyfat and keep it off because muscle has a higher resting metabolic rate than fat. Muscle tissue is highly active even when it is resting, whereas fat tissue is comparitively inactive.[2] A higher constant metabolic rate is a great way to get rid of unwanted fat. This factor works for you all of the time – on days off and even when you sleep! Increasing your metabolic rate is a super-slick way to a slim, shapely body.

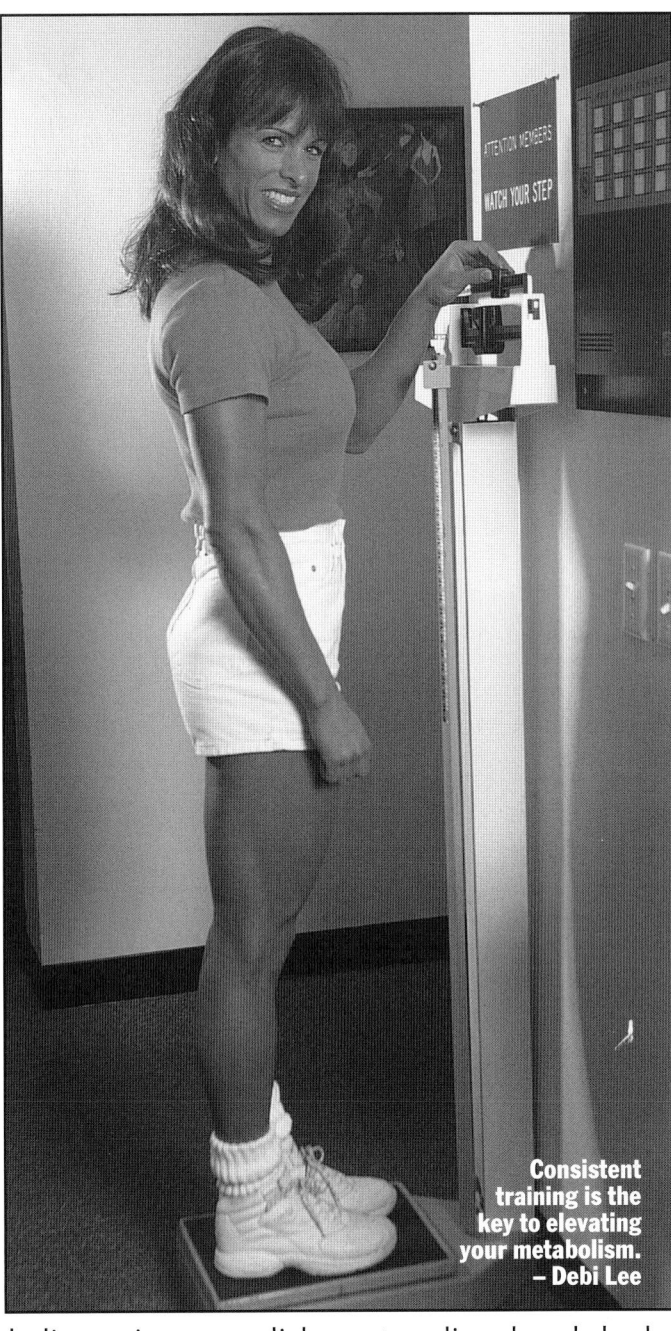

Consistent training is the key to elevating your metabolism.
– Debi Lee

Weightlifting

The key to elevating your metabolism is training on a consistent basis, utilizing a weightlifting program. An occasional lifting session is not enough – your body needs a constant challenge to stay in top muscle-toned condition.

CHAPTER TWO

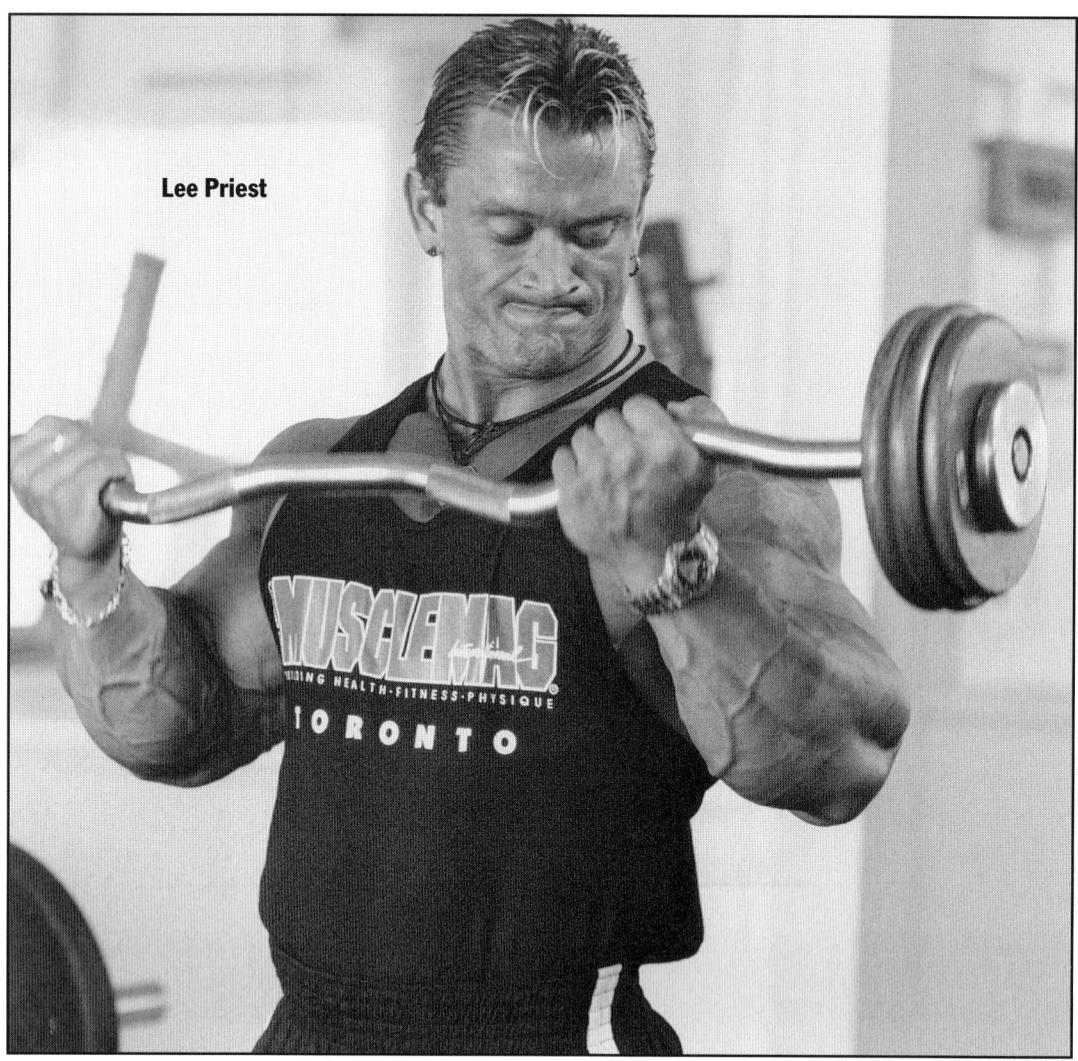

Lee Priest

On the other hand, a consistent weightlifting approach does not mean lifting weights every day. In fact, lifting weights too often can be detrimental to your body. The best approach is to get in a couple of weight-training workouts per week, and to make sure you exercise each major muscle group one or two times a week, every week. Working your major muscle groups less than once a week is insufficient while more than twice a week may cause overtraining and lead to injuries. The same muscle group should not be worked two days in a row, but should receive a 48-hour rest before being trained again.

The first step in the *Metabolic Magic* course for carving off fat is to train with weights on a consistent basis. If you have not been lifting weights it is time to start; if you have only lifted weights on occassion, it is time to make weight training an essential part of your physique-shaping program.

Metabolic Magic

Step One
- Start lifting weights on a regular basis.
- Allow at least 48 hours rest between weightlifting workouts that train the same muscle group.
- Work the larger muscle groups (chest, back, legs).

That's all there is to Step One!

Checklist
- Have you started lifting weights at home, or at a local gym, health club, or a friend's place?
- Are you training the major muscle groups in your workout?
- Are you training both your upper and lower body at least once per week?
- Are you giving each muscle group at least 48 hours of rest before working it again?
- Are you working out on a consistent basis?

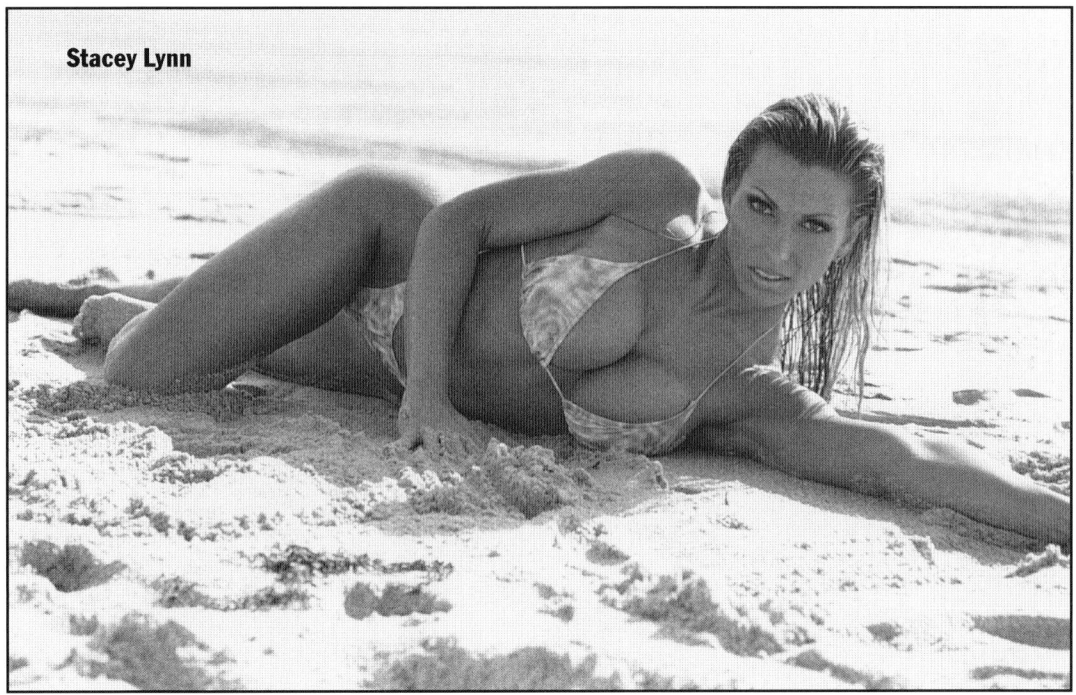
Stacey Lynn

References
1. Eva May Hamilton & Eleanor Whitney, *Nutrition: Concepts and Controversies* (New York: West Publishing Company, 1979), 215.
2. Hamilton & Whitney, *Nutrition*, 156.

CHAPTER THREE

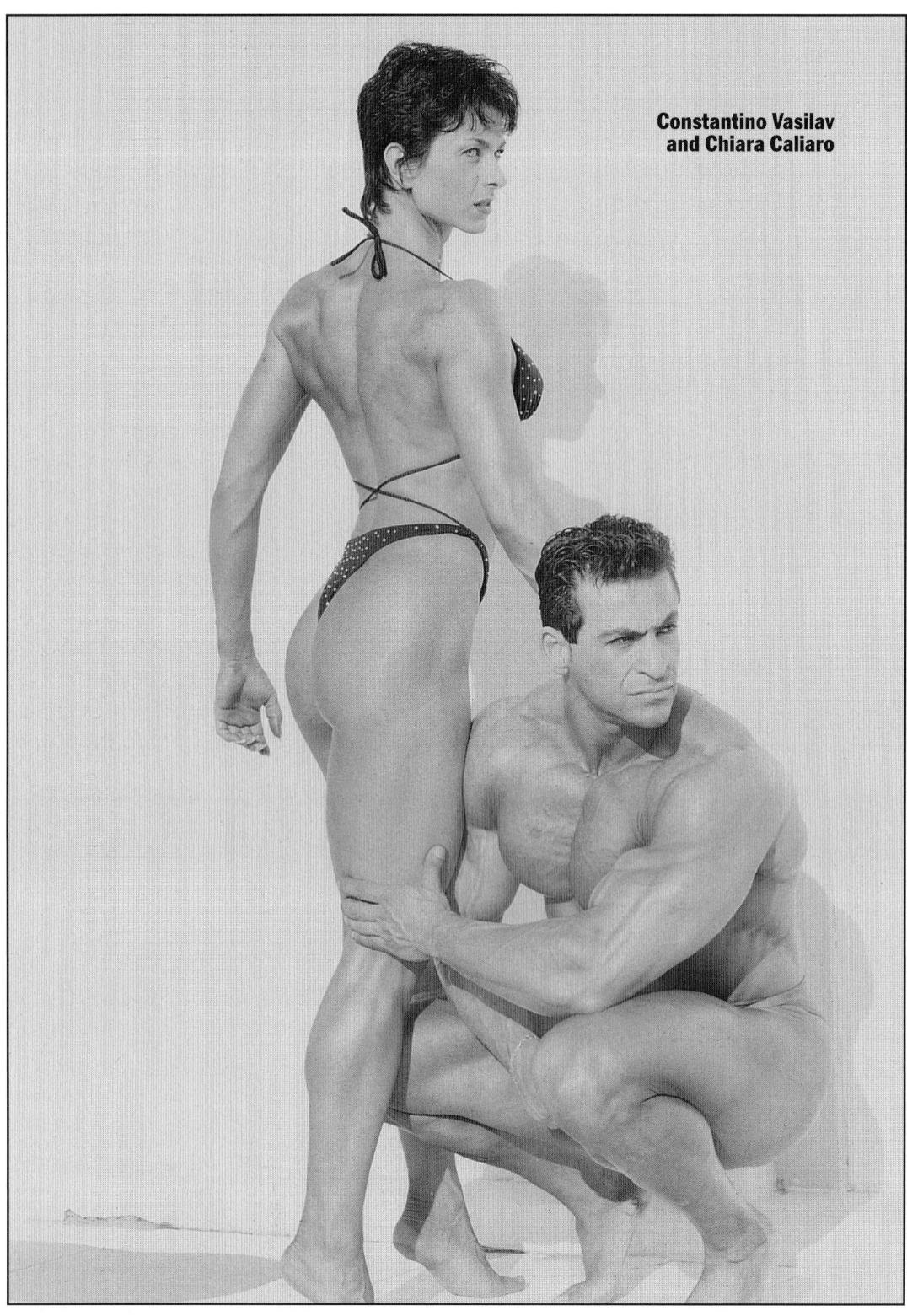

Constantino Vasilav and Chiara Caliaro

Fighting Fat: Cutting Carbs

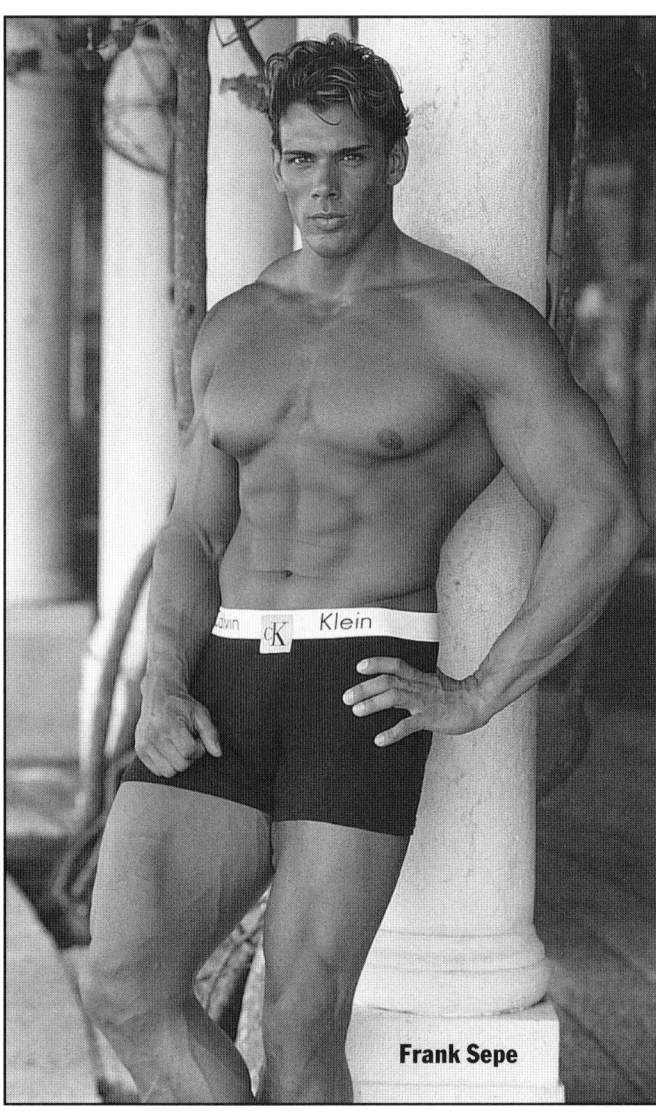

Frank Sepe

When most people think of burning off bodyfat they think of restricting their fat intake. A lower fat intake can help prevent you from gaining unwanted bodyweight. But avoiding fat is not the only dietary adjustment that you can make. The *Metabolic Magic* program contains another fat-loss technique that works very well for getting rid of bodyfat – decreasing your intake of carbohydrates.

Great Fat-Reduction Technique

At one time, athletes who were concerned with the appearance of their physiques didn't pay much attention to what they ate. However, as the sport of bodybuilding progressed, many found that what they ate made a significant difference in their appearance. One of the bodybuilders who excelled during this time was Frank Zane, a champion during the pioneer phase of physique training. Zane, a multiple Mr. Olympia winner, was well-known

CHAPTER THREE

for his fantastically symmetrical and low-fat physique. One of the techniques he used was to drastically lower his carb intake. Frank's diet consisted of lots of meat, an abundance of oils (the healthy fats) and very little carbohydrates, but he did include some vegetables. Zane pointed out that before he went to the low-carbohydrate diet he was pretty smooth. He discovered that the best manner in which to trim down was to eat the minimum amount of carbohydrates required without going into ketosis. Zane said that when you go into ketosis (from a zero-carbohydrate diet) you "lose muscle mass, so you need enough carbohydrates to stay out of ketosis but not too much more."[1]

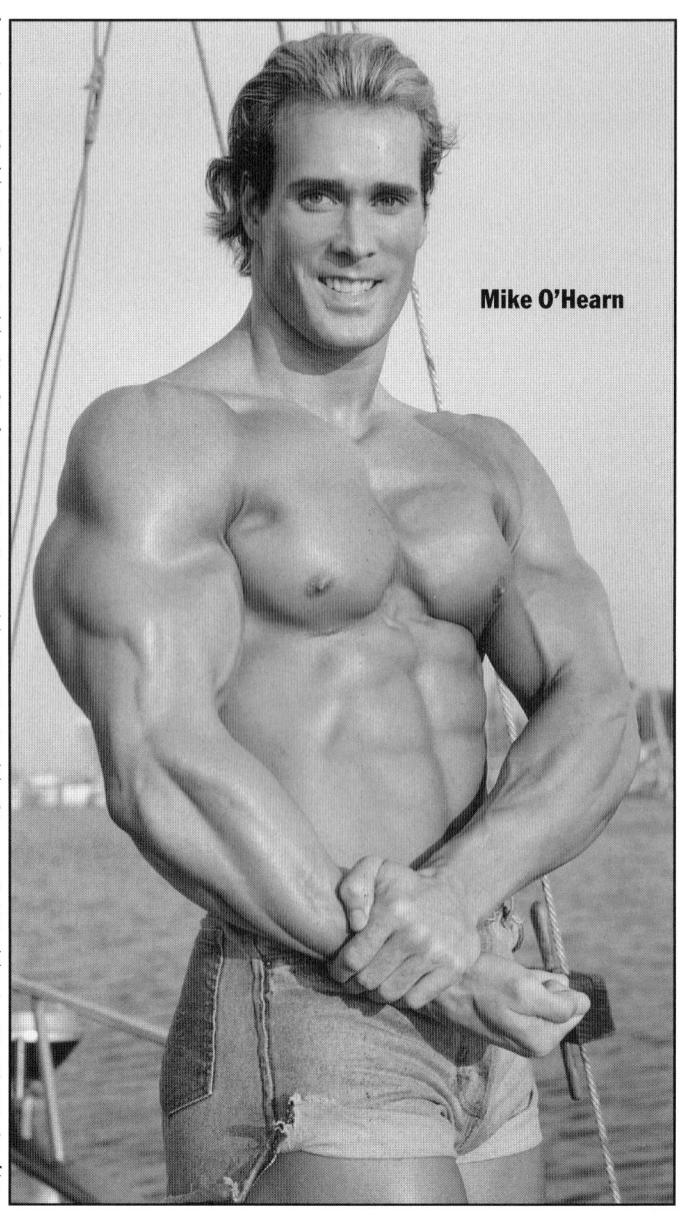

Mike O'Hearn

Significantly lowering your carbohydrate intake is a great technique for burning off bodyfat. Many people get hung up on lowering their fat intake without realizing that carbohydrates can also make you fat, particularly when you eat too many per meal. Fat is not the primary factor for unwanted weight gain problems. Excess carbohydrate caloric intake, particularly in the area of simple carbohydrates (sugar types) can add up quickly, and weight gain is inevitable. Fitness and dietary expert Jay Robb points out that "if you are eating a high-carb diet and are not in constant motion, there is a good chance many of those extra carbohydrates will join together and become love handles."[2] Most people are not active enough to burn off all the extra carbohydrates they ingest.

When you eat carbohydrates they get converted into glucose and they must be burned quickly or it turns into bodyfat. Excess carbohydrates do not evaporate – they turn into fat. And once bodyfat gets a foothold on your physique it is hard to get rid of. What is the solution? Quite simple – lower your intake of carbohydrates. The less carbohydrates you have available to turn to bodyfat, the less fat that gets stored on your physique.

And the absence of excess carbohydrates in the diet is not the only factor involved in this approach to fat loss. There is a second factor as well. The first factor is that a lower carbohydrate intake means there is less excess carbohydrates to be turned to fat. The second factor is that when there is not a lot of carbohydrates for the body to use as fuel, the body turns to fat as the fuel source.

The lower carbohydrate diet is a very effective fat trimming tool. It has two factors working in its favor – the lack of available carbohydrates for use as a main fuel source prevents the body from taking those carbohydrates and storing them as fat, and it also causes the body to switch over to using the unwanted fat that the body does have as a fuel source – as the primary fuel source.

Low Carb, not No Carb

A low carbohydrate diet means just that – a low carbohydrate intake, not a total absence of carbohydrates. Your body needs some carbohydrates as fuel for action, particularly for shape/strength workouts. And going too low on the carbohydrate intake can cause ketosis, which is an undesirable state where your muscles are eaten up by the body as fuel. Also, it is especially important that a pregnant woman does not go on a low-carbohydrate diet.

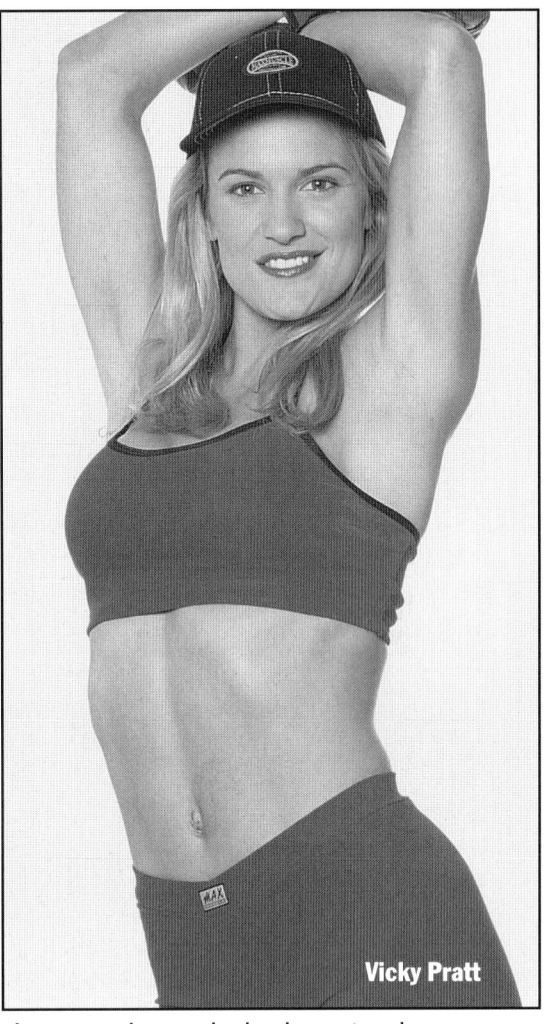

Another point – don't always use a low-carbohydrate diet approach. Switch at times to a higher carbohydrate intake. Use the low carbohydrate approach in cyclical fashion – use it for a long period, then switch to a higher carbohydrate diet for a while, and then once again go back to the lower carbohydrate intake. Variety works as well with the diet as it does in other areas.

As has been pointed out, some carbohydrates are necessary. The totally no-carbohydrate diets are not a good idea. The best approach is with a moderate amount of carbohydrate intake, taking more before and directly after a workout, and less during the rest of the week.

Vicky Pratt

CHAPTER THREE

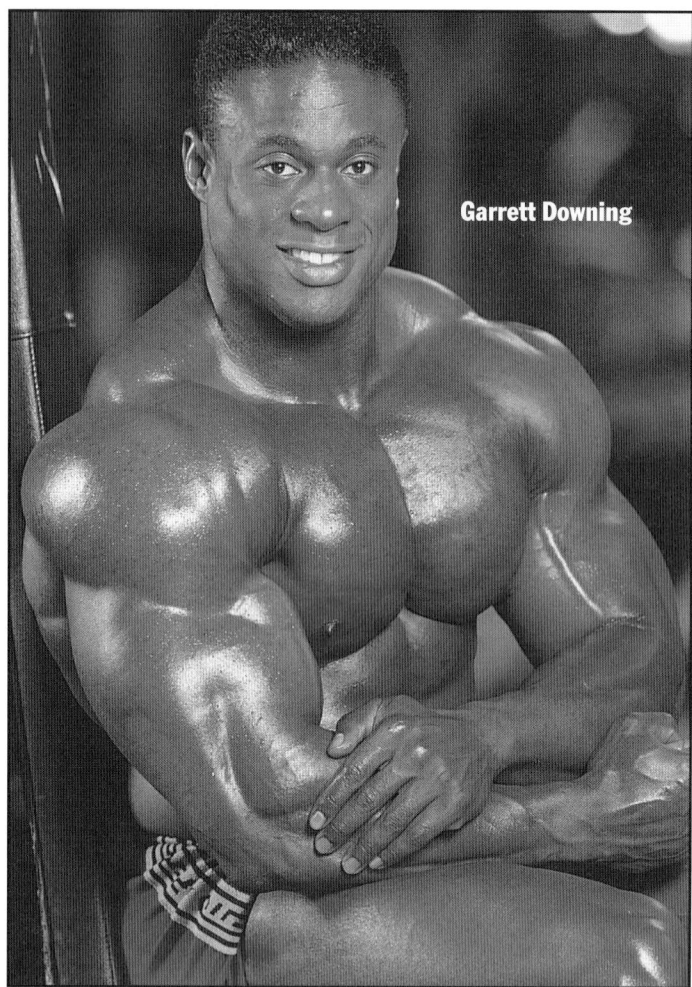

Garrett Downing

Sources

The best carbohydrate sources are those that are full of fiber (vegetables, oats, grains, beans, etc.) and are considered complex carbohydrates. These types of carbohydrates burn off at a slower and smoother rate and keep your insulin level at a more even level. The undesirable carbohydrates are the simple carbohydrates. These types of carbohydrates hit your body in a highly concentrated and active form that spikes your insulin level way up, then drops it back down, and takes it even lower than where you were before ingesting the simple carbs. These types of carbs are the most prone to pack on the excess bodyfat to your physique. Eat a moderately low amount of carbohydrates from the best sources (complex and fibrous) and avoid the simple carbohydrates as much as possible. The one time that you want to take some simple carbohydrates is about one and a half hours before a shape/strength workout and within one and a half hours after a strength/shape workout. Beside that time, avoid the simple carbohydrates like the plague, and don't eat too much complex carbohydrates. The second simple step for the *Metabolic Magic* program is to lower your carbohydrate intake.

Step Two

- Lower your carbohydrate intake.
- Gradually cut out the excess carbohydrates in your diet until you begin to see a noticeable decrease in your bodyfat levels. Stay at this level of carbohydrate intake.
- Cut out most simple carbohydrate intake except for 1 1/2 hours before and after a shape/strength workout.
- Low carbohydrate does not mean no carbohydrate – eat some carbohydrates each day to avoid ketosis.

Metabolic Magic

Checklist

Have you:
- Started to gradually cut back on your carbohydrate intake?
- Started reading food labels to find out how many carbohydrate grams each serving contains?
- Are you checking for the amount of simple sugars in the food you eat and specifically avoiding them?
- Are you eating some carbohydrates (and avoiding the too-low carbohydrate diet)?
- Are you starting to substitute fresh foods for fast foods and junk food? Eating at home more often – at least once more per week than currently?

References
1. Bill Dobbins, Pioneering Diets, FLEX, May 1996, p. 102
2. Ibid

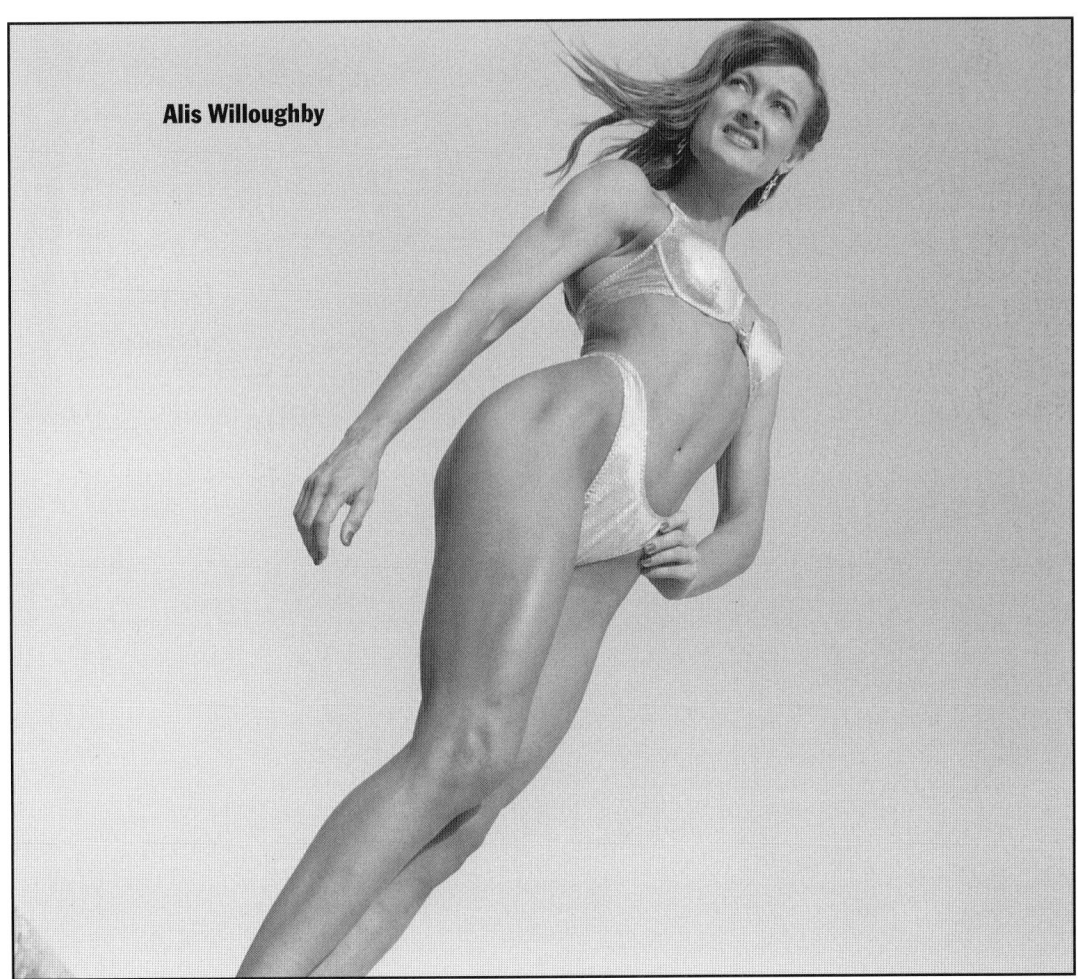

Alis Willoughby

CHAPTER FOUR

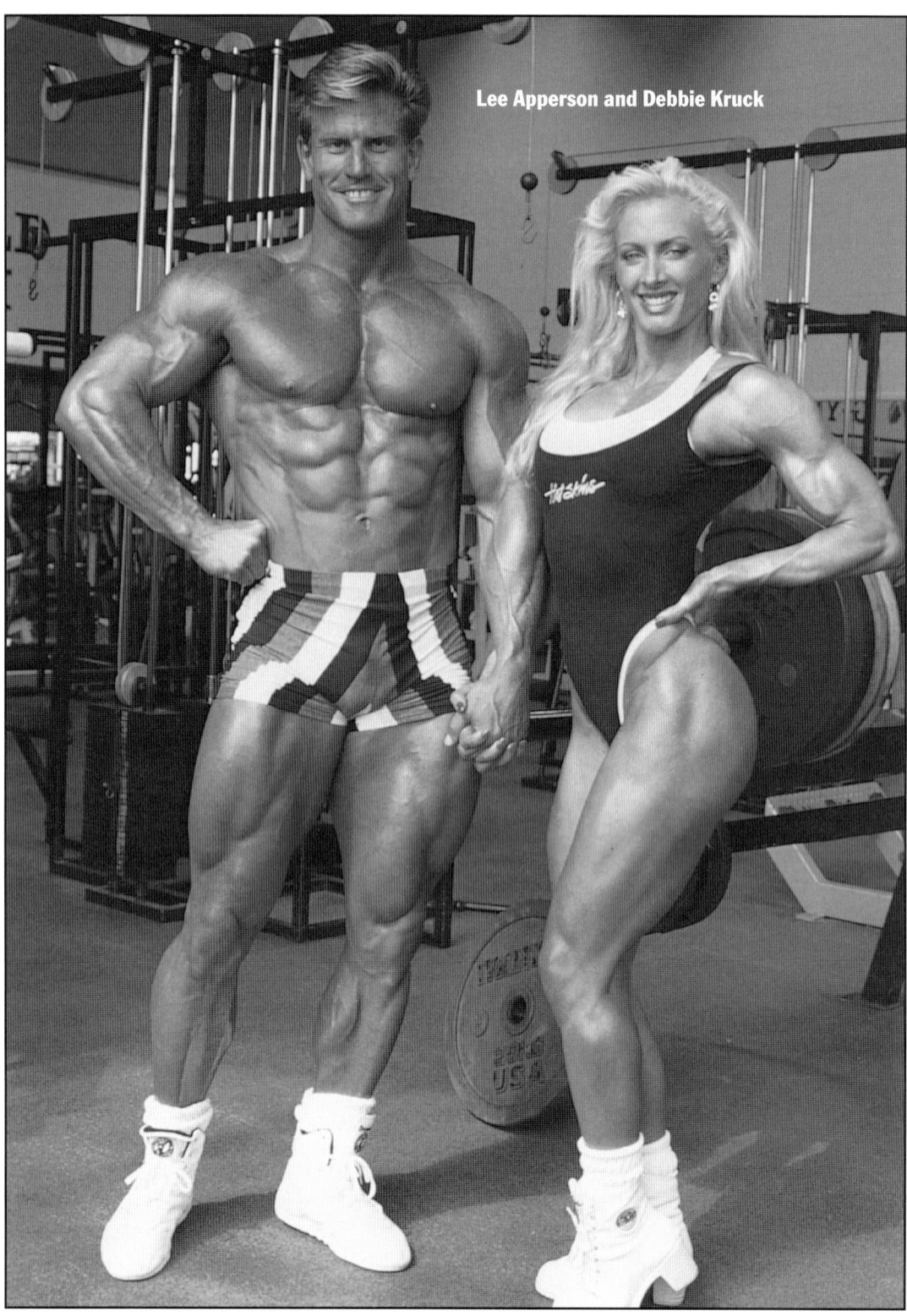

Lee Apperson and Debbie Kruck

Fiber for Fat

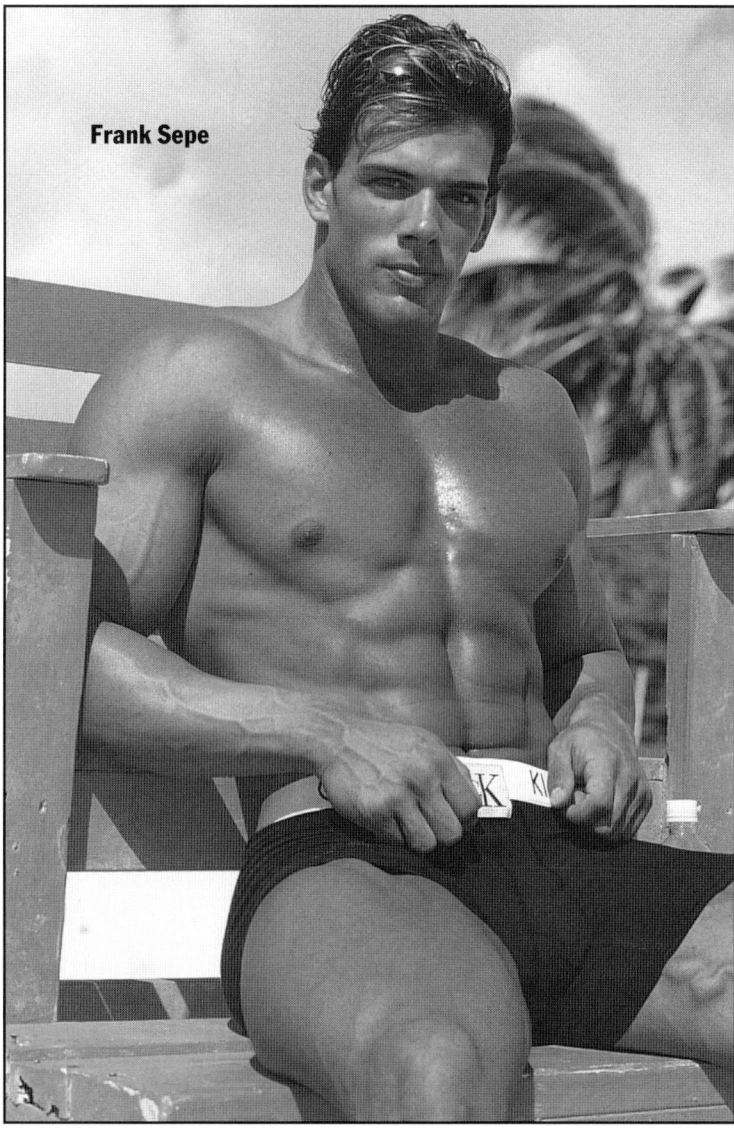

Frank Sepe

With a reduction in simple carbs, your body will begin to crave them. Your best defence in the battle of the bulge is fiber.

Heavy Hitter

Fat is no lightweight when it comes to calories. Fat contains more than twice as much caloric value per gram as either protein or carbohydrates. Protein and carbohydrates do not go directly on to the physique as fat; only excess amounts of protein or carbohydrates are converted into fat. Fat, on the other hand, goes directly onto the body as fat.

A small amount of fat is necessary for most body functions. Without any fat intake your body would soon develop major problems. However, beyond the small amount that the body needs, excess fat has no real function. Excess bodyfat hinders the body in its movements and health, and it looks unattractive to most people. People recognize this and go to all kinds of lengths to get rid of unwanted fat. They starve themselves, go on fad diets, buy new exercise equipment and do many other such strange things to beat the problem of bodyfat.

CHAPTER FOUR

Fiber for Fat

The basic idea behind exchanging fiber for fat is to cut back on your fat intake and replace the excess calories from fat with fibrous foods. What does this do? It really helps the body in many ways. Too much fat causes health problems while more fiber helps solve health problems. But there is more involved than just that – fiber in exchange of fat helps in a variety of manners. When it comes to fiber intake, both soluble and especially insoluble, there is a slight boost in your metabolic action (in order for these more bulky foods to be digested/eliminated) from fiber intake. Dietary fiber is resistant to hydrolysis by human digestive enzymes. This causes a slight increase in metabolic activity as the body handles the fat. The indigestible bulk in the stomach is what the muscles of the intestines exercise against, and this exercising can cause a small increase in metabolic activity.

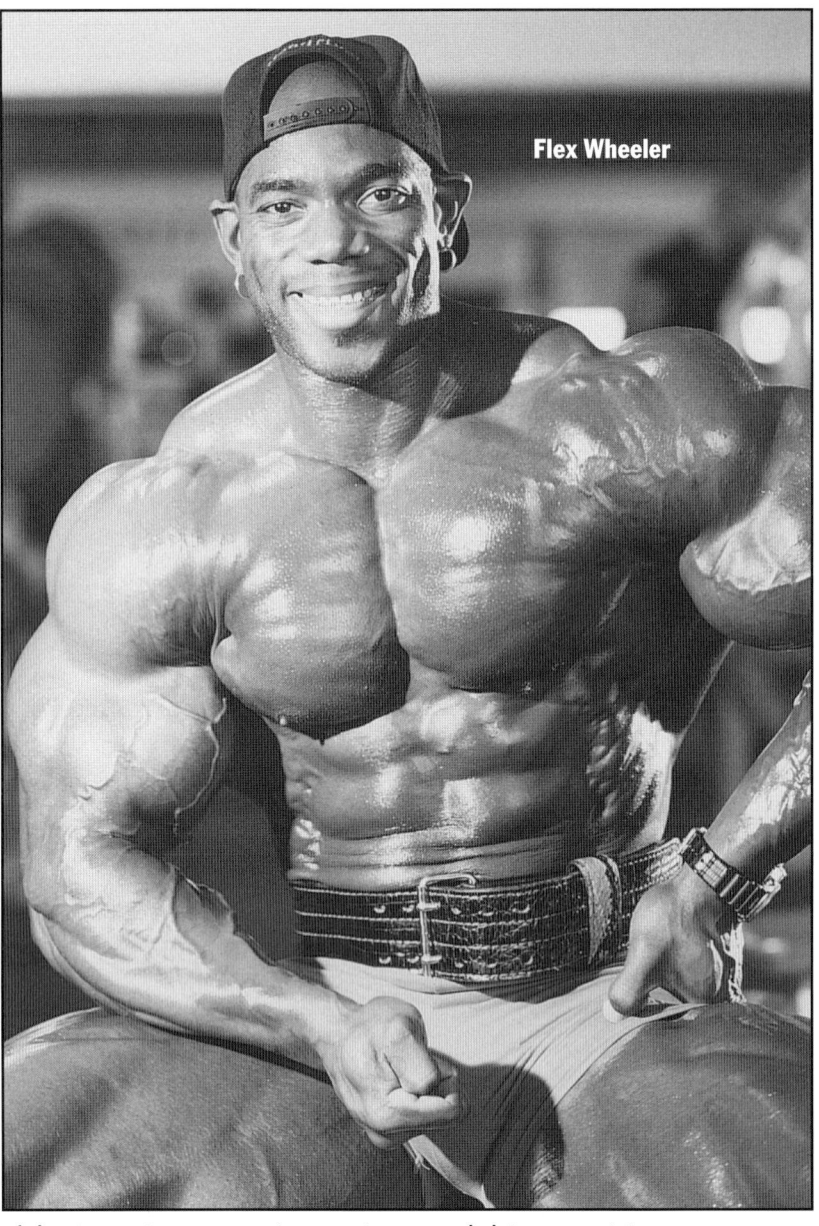

Flex Wheeler

    The fiber for fat exchange is fantastic in several ways – you are exchanging the high calorie food (fat) for a low calorie food (fiber). You are exchanging a food that is easily digested and turns readily into fat for one that is not easily digested (the process of fiber activity also slightly heats up the metabolism) and does not turn into fat at all. And you are exchanging a food, fat, which has 9 calories per gram, for a food that has no calories per gram, a 9 for 0 exchange.

Metabolic Magic

Sources

The best sources of soluble fiber are oat bran, beans, barley and lentils. The best sources of insoluble fibers are wheat bran, corn bran, peas and seeds.

Among cereals, many of the "bran" cereals are very high in fiber. Among fruits, apples, raisins, dried prunes, figs, pear (with skin), oranges and strawberries are high in fiber. In vegetables, potatoes (with skin), broccoli and carrots have a high fiber content. Celery is another good source of fiber (which has a lot of insoluble fiber). So are spinach, tomatoes, cabbage and lettuce. Nuts, popcorn and seeds have a good amount of fiber in them as well.

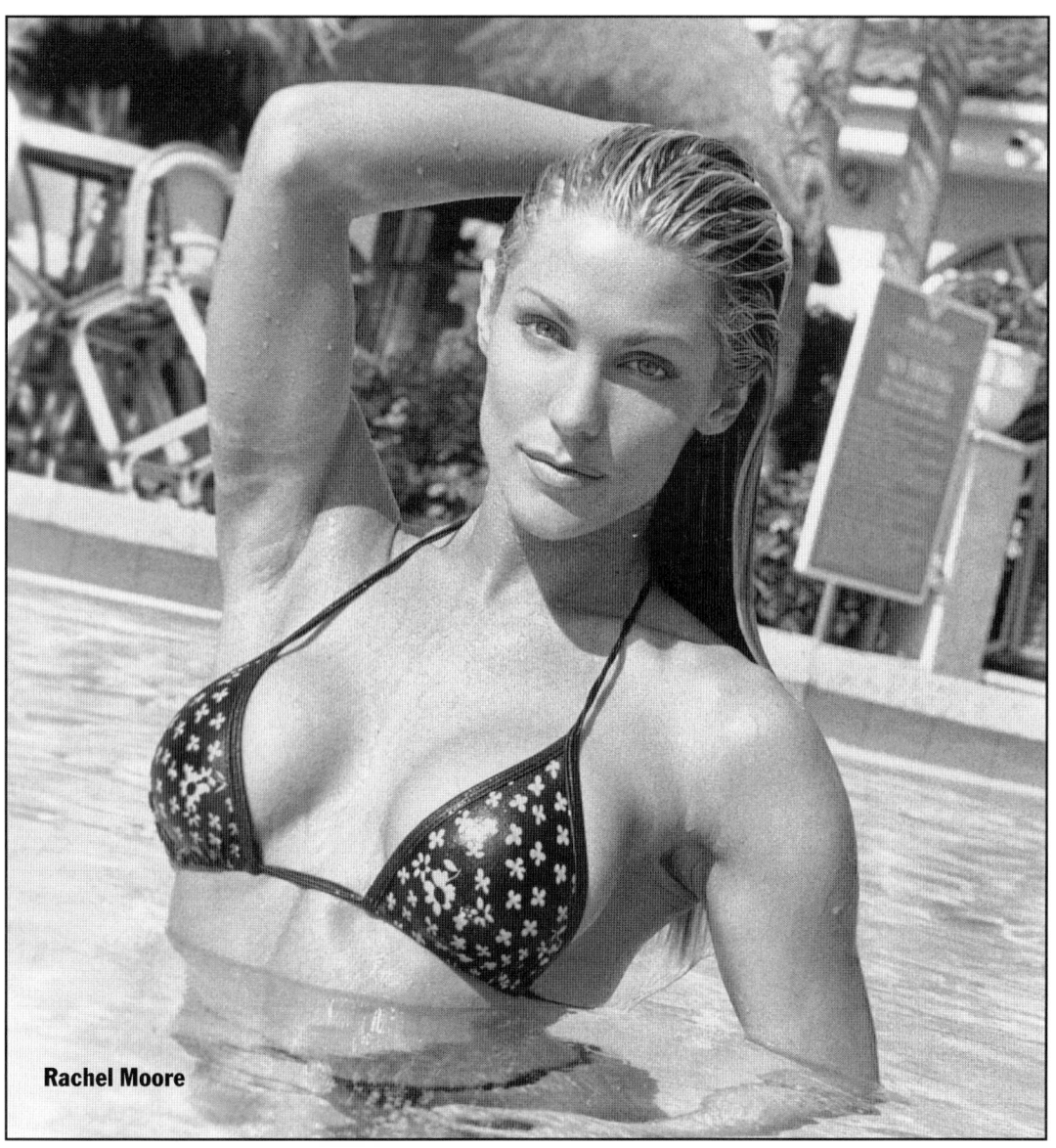
Rachel Moore

CHAPTER FOUR

Don't Go Overboard

As good as fiber is for you, you can get too much of a good thing when it comes to this substance. Consuming very large amounts of fiber (50+ grams a day) can deplete your body of essential vitamins and minerals. A better range is 20-35 grams of fiber every day. This is more than most people take and often takes a conscious effort to achieve. But if you focus on the foods mentioned previously (that have more fiber than most) you can get your daily fiber dose. Also check the back panel on packaged food items. The ingredient list will identify what types of food elements are in the food (protein, carbohydrates, fat) and how much is included in each serving. Check the various food items that you buy to ensure that you are getting enough fiber on a daily basis.

Fiber Tips

There are a few things that you can do to include a larger amount of fiber in your diet.
- Avoid refined foods as much as possible. The refinement process often deletes fiber from the food.
- Eat vegetables and fruit in a raw or near-raw state (lightly steamed).
- Eat mostly whole-grain cereals instead of refined cereals (most hot cereals are not refined and contain little or no sugar).

You can increase your fiber intake if you are careful in selecting the foods that you eat. There are many positive reasons to increase your fiber intake – fiber helps you in living a more healthy lifestyle, and it helps you in controlling the appearance of your physique. You can double the effectiveness of this action by exchanging fat intake for fiber intake. Of course you need a little fat, but beyond a small amount, you can substitute fibrous foods for fatty foods. Doing so will help your physique look much better. Step four of the *Metabolic Magic* program is to exchange fiber for fat – to replace the fat in your diet with foods that are high in fiber.

Step Three

- Cut out most (not all) of the fatty foods from your diet.
- Greatly increase your intake of fiber (20-35 grams a day).
- Eat both soluble and insoluble fiber.

Checklist

Have you:
- Reduced your fat intake?
- Increased your fiber intake?
- Are you getting a good amount of both soluble and insoluble fiber?

Metabolic Magic

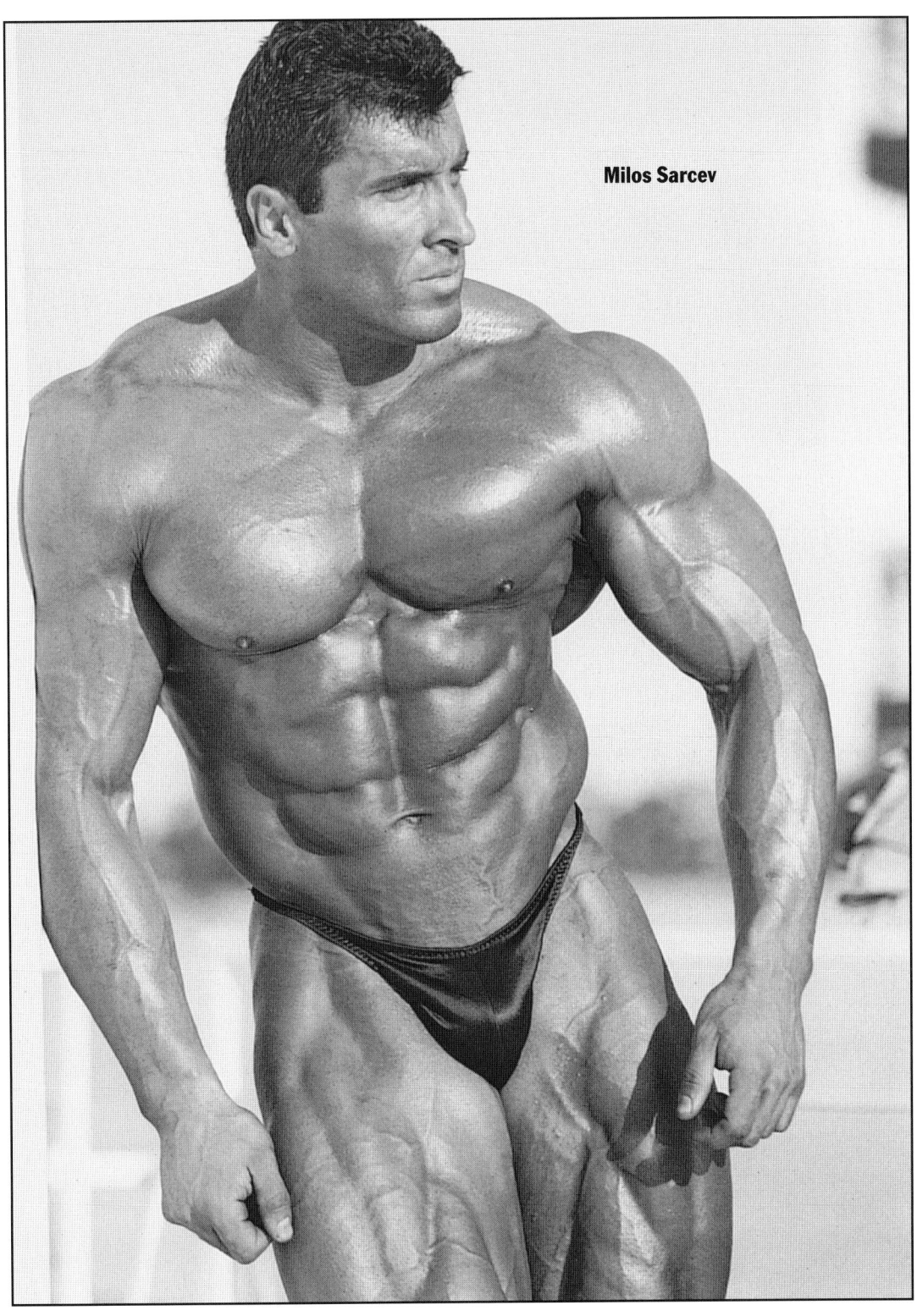

Milos Sarcev

CHAPTER FIVE

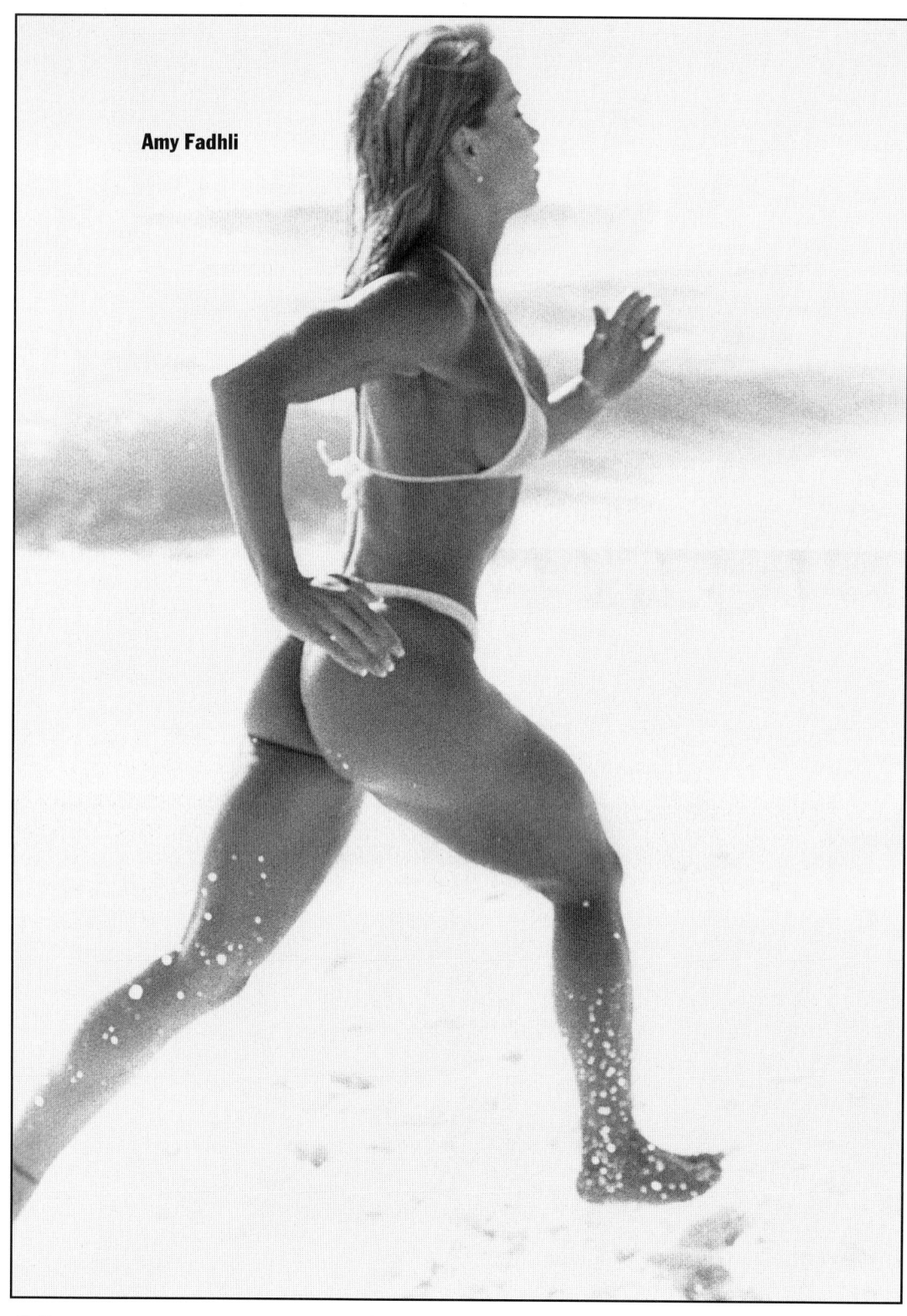

Long and Moderate Cardio/aerobic Workouts

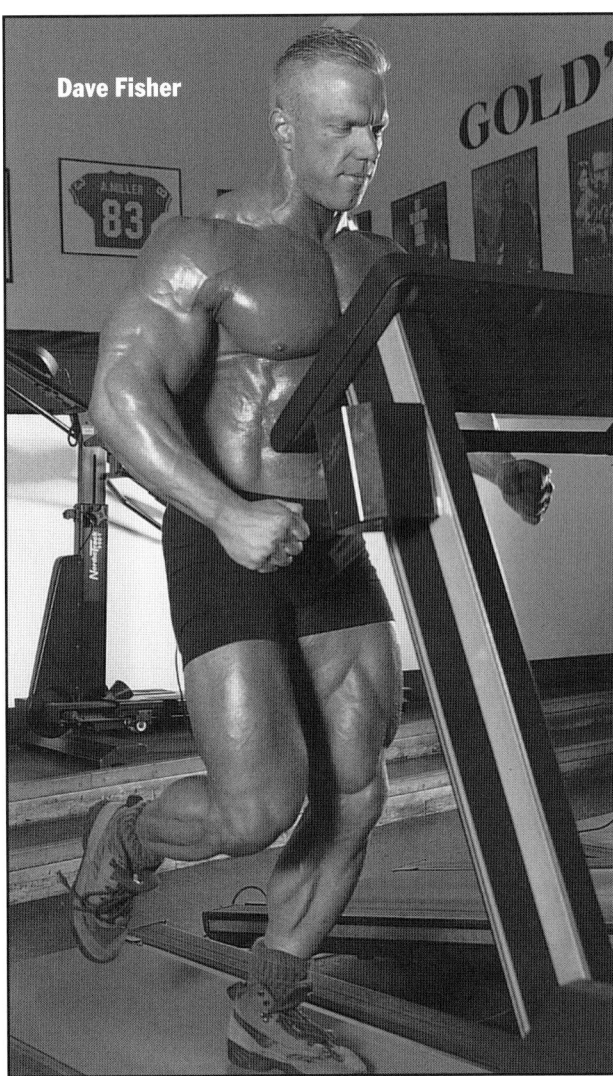

Dave Fisher

Cardiovascular/aerobic workouts are another very good tool to use to burn off bodyfat if they are used correctly. The manner in which you use a cardio/aerobic workout is crucial for getting all of the fat-burning benefits possible. This means first knowing how to use cardio/aerobic training in a way that translates into a loss of bodyfat, and then using that approach to get rid of your bodyfat. The very best manner in which to burn off bodyfat with cardio/aerobic workouts is with a longer and moderate workout.

Fast and Furious Futility

Many people tend to approach their cardio/aerobic workouts with the attitude of getting the job done as quickly as possible. Their workout pace is fast and furious. They may run a quick mile or two, or they may dash up all the stairs at

CHAPTER FIVE

work instead of taking the elevator. The pace that they use is rapid. The problem is that a rapid pace is not necessarily the best for burning off bodyfat. In fact, the best pace for burning off bodyfat is a more moderate pace.

You burn more fat as a percentage of all fuel consumed in low intensity exercise as compared to high intensity exercise. When someone jumps on an exercise machine and goes all-out for several minutes, all they are doing is burning up their immediate glycogen storage. And the faster and more furious they go, the more likely they are to be using glycogen as fuel than fat as the fuel source. Burning calories and burning fat are not necessarily the same thing! A more moderate pace is more likely to cause the body to use fat as the fuel source. The best way to use fat for fuel during a workout is with a cardio/aerobic workout that utilizes a longer time frame and a more moderate pace.

Longer Session

The longer cardio/aerobic session is better for removing bodyfat for several reasons. As has been mentioned, the longer you workout the more fat you use as fuel – you use only a little fat for a fuel source initially, but gradually use more and more fat for a percentage of the fuel as you continue to workout. There is also the factor of the "post-workout" effect. Of course this is greatest in strength/shape workouts, but it also does play a factor in cardio/aerobic workouts.

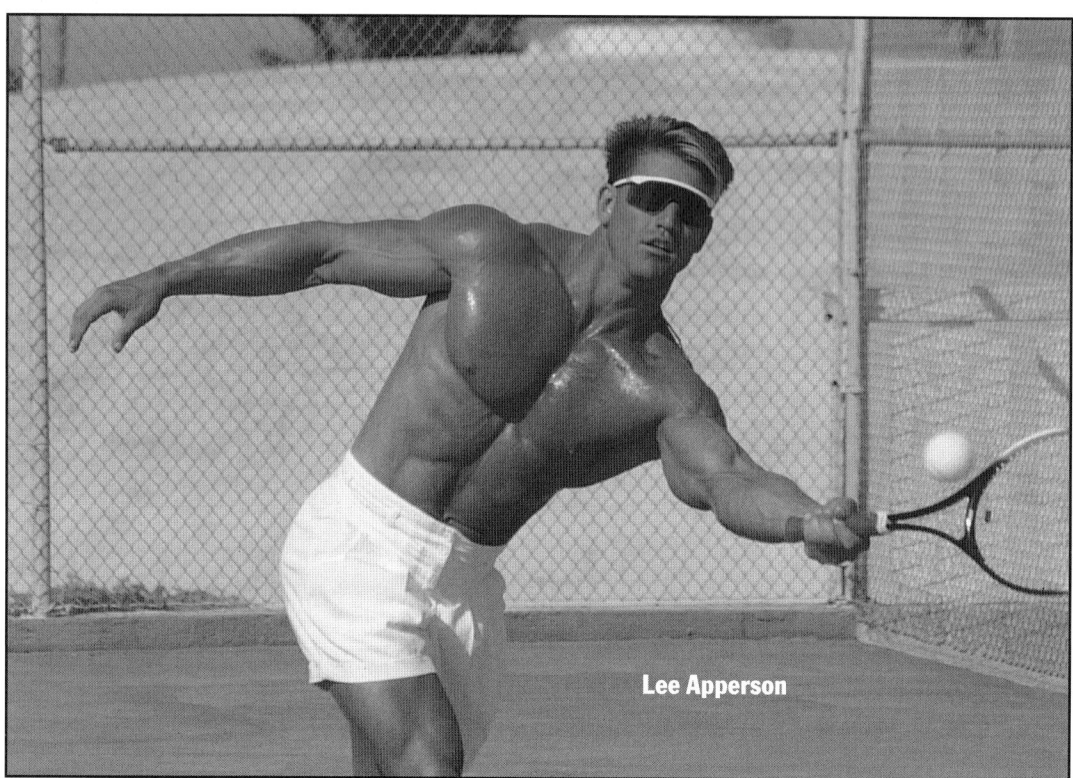
Lee Apperson

28

Metabolic Magic

The post-workout caloric burn (of fat) is much more effective from a longer workout than from a shorter workout. Simply put, a longer workout is a better fat burning tool.

Gradually Build Up

Although the best manner in which to burn off fat during an exercise session is with a longer workout, it is not the best idea to immediately jump into a super-long workout mode. Gradually build up to a longer workout session. If you normally perform 20 to 30 minutes of cardio/aerobic work, add five minutes at your next workout, and then another five minutes at the following workout. Increase your workout time frame by steps instead of in one instant leap. This will be more beneficial for the health of your physique and also let your mind (which plays a very large part in sustaining you through a longer routine) become accustomed to the idea of the longer workout. So get to the longer workouts via an incremental process instead of an instant process.

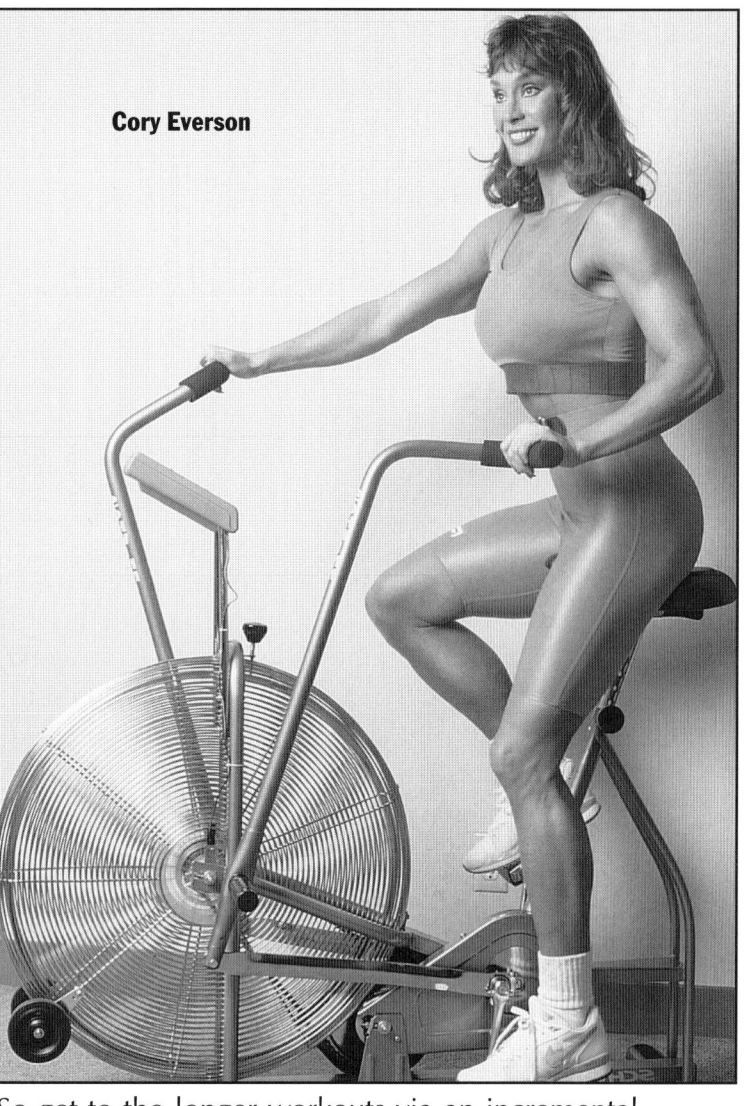
Cory Everson

Pace

What rate should you be performing your longer workout at? The best rate is a rate of approximately 55 to 70 percent of your maximum heart rate (MHR). If you go too far beyond this range you will tend to use more glycogen as your fuel source instead of fat. And if you are below this suggested rate (55 percent to 70 percent) you will not give your body enough of a challenge to stimulate much fuel burning at all. Aim at working out at a moderate pace, which equates to the 55 to 70 percent of MHR. The *Metabolic Magic* program pace for cardio/aerobic workouts is 55 percent to 70 percent of MHR.

CHAPTER FIVE

Step Four

- Perform a longer cardio/aerobic exercise routine.
- Gradually work up to the longer routine.
- Perform the routine at a more moderate pace (55 to 70 percent of maximum heart rate).

Checklist

Have you:
- Made a commitment to start getting in longer cardiovascular/aerobic workouts?
- Gradually increased the length of the cardio/aerobic workout?
- Performed your cardio/aerobic workouts at a moderate pace (as opposed to a fast and furious pace)?

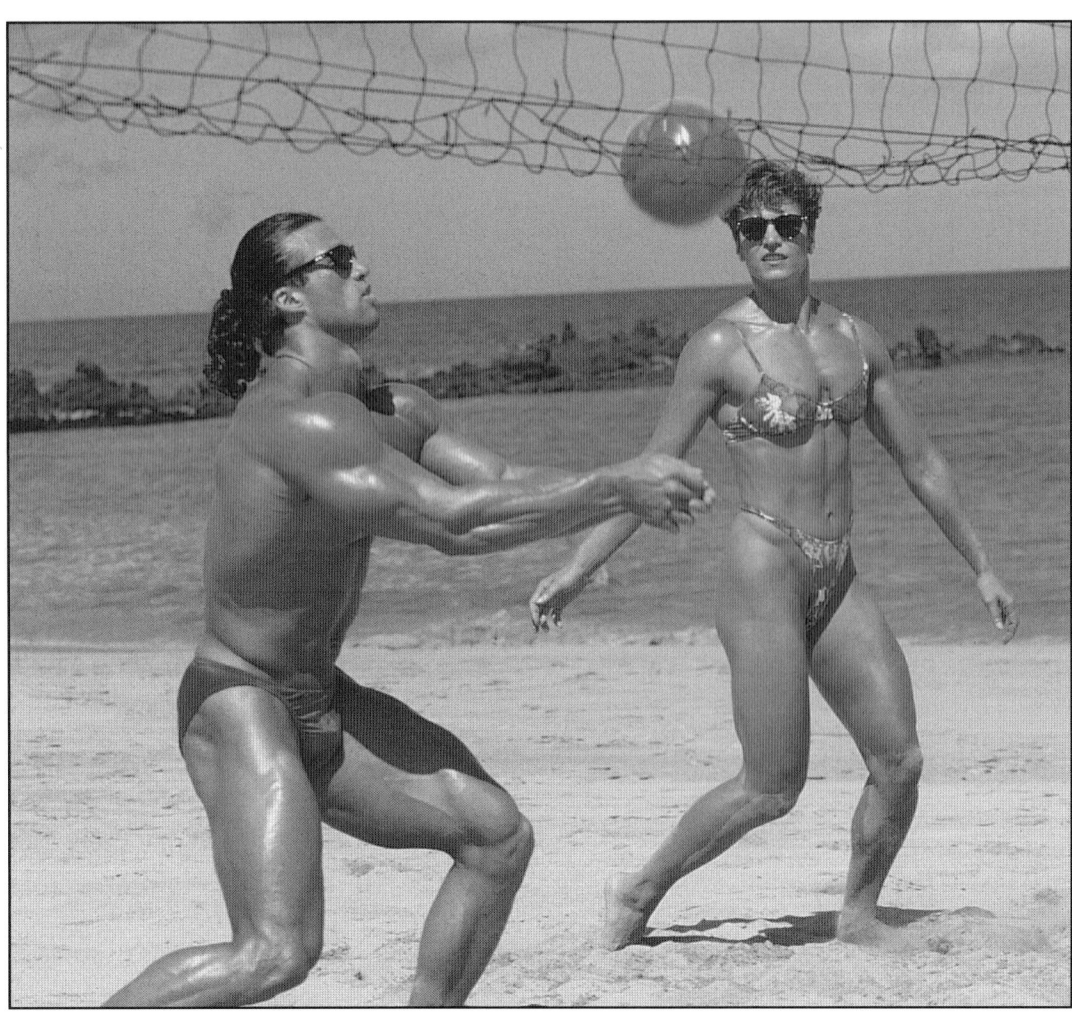

Metabolic Magic

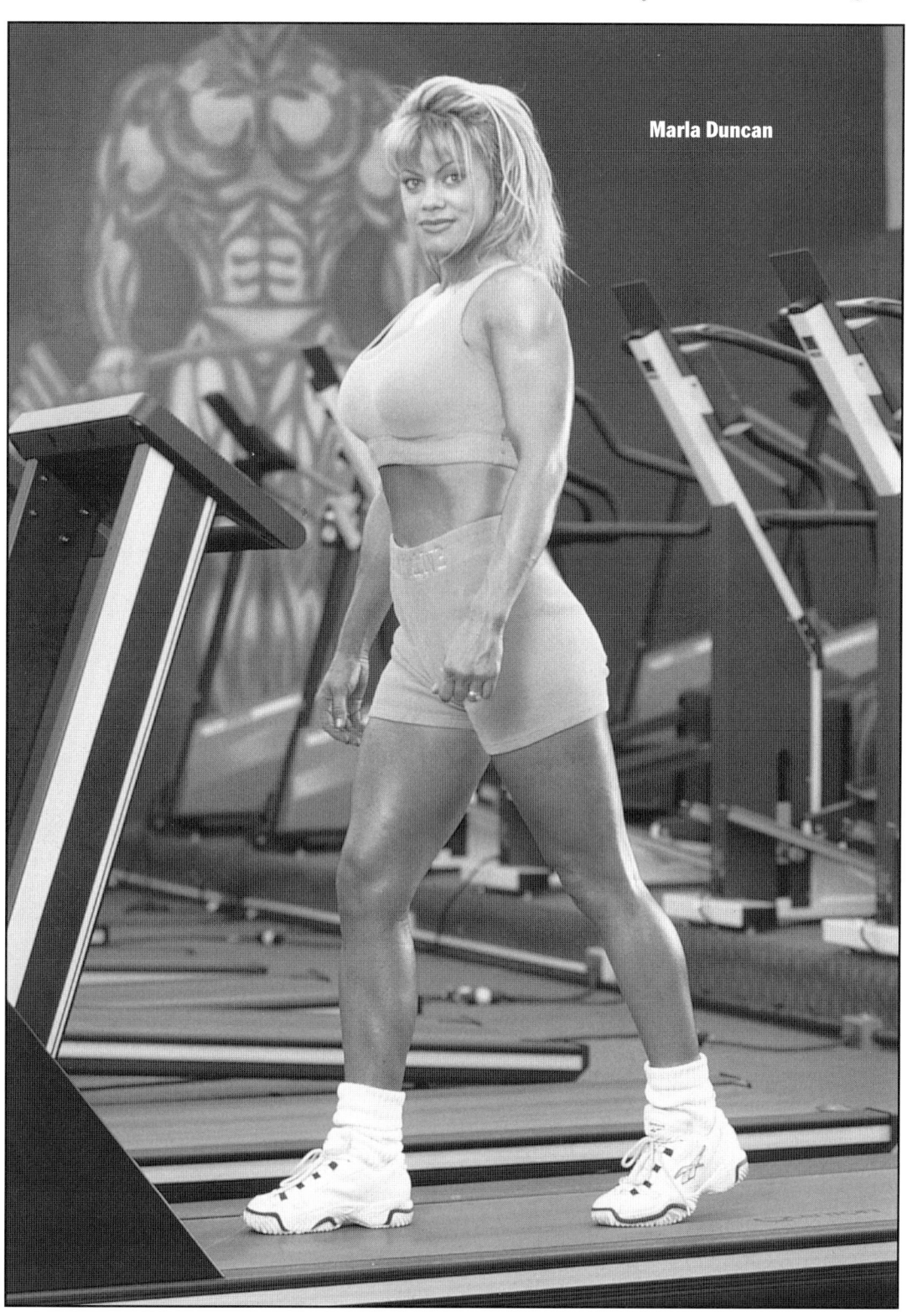

Marla Duncan

CHAPTER SIX

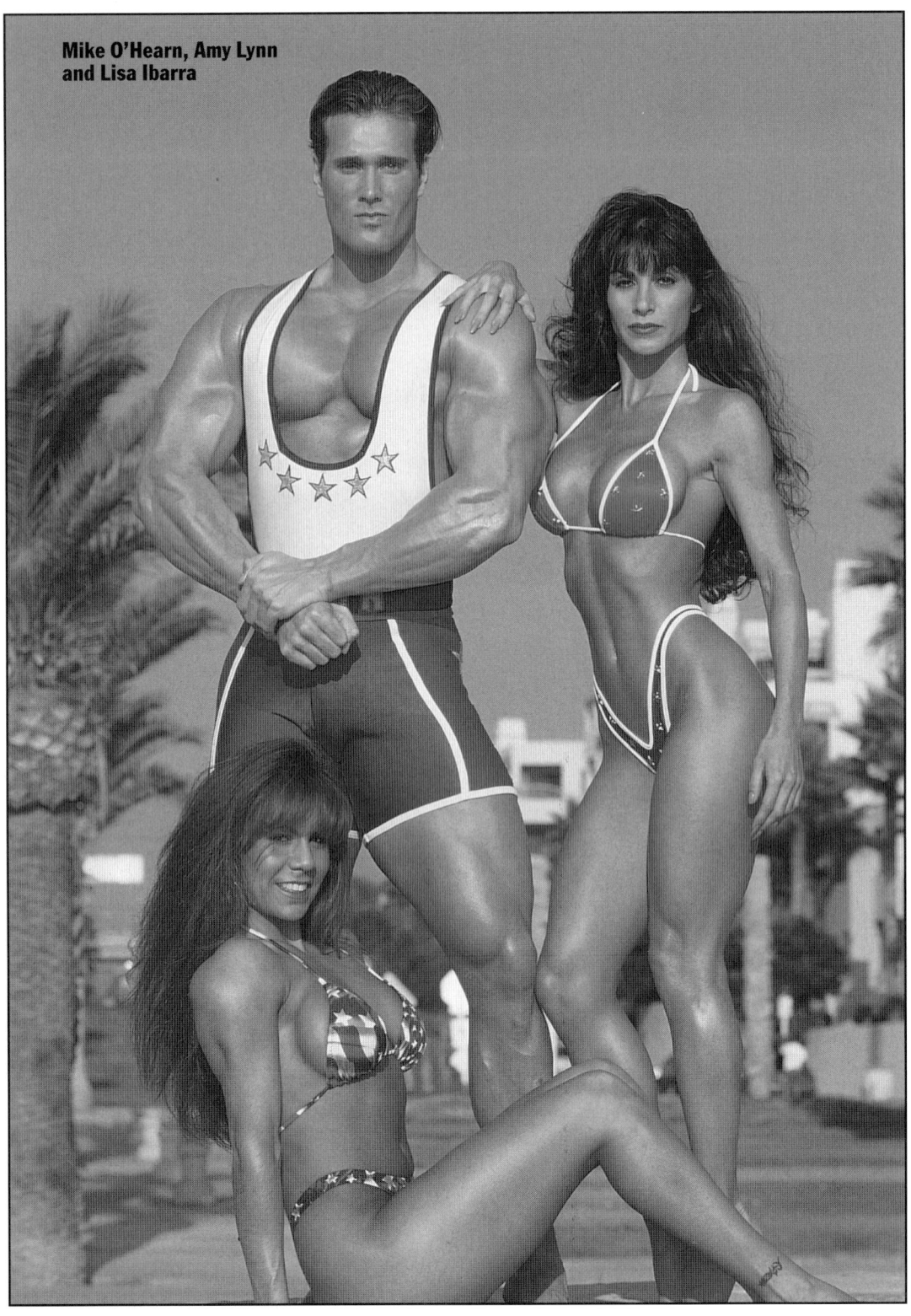

Mike O'Hearn, Amy Lynn and Lisa Ibarra

The Metabolic Program

The *Metabolic Magic* program consists of just four basic steps: weightlifting for weight loss, cutting back on carbohydrate intake, longer and more moderate cardio/aerobic workouts, and exchanging fiber for fat. Each of these steps are important and essential to the overall goal – of making your physique more slender. Any one of the steps works well, but when combined the four steps create magic – the magic of a slender shape.

Your metabolism plays a very important role in getting rid of bodyfat, and preventing any unwanted bodyfat from accumulating. The *Metabolic Magic* program utilizesyour body metabolism as a weapon in the war on fat. By using

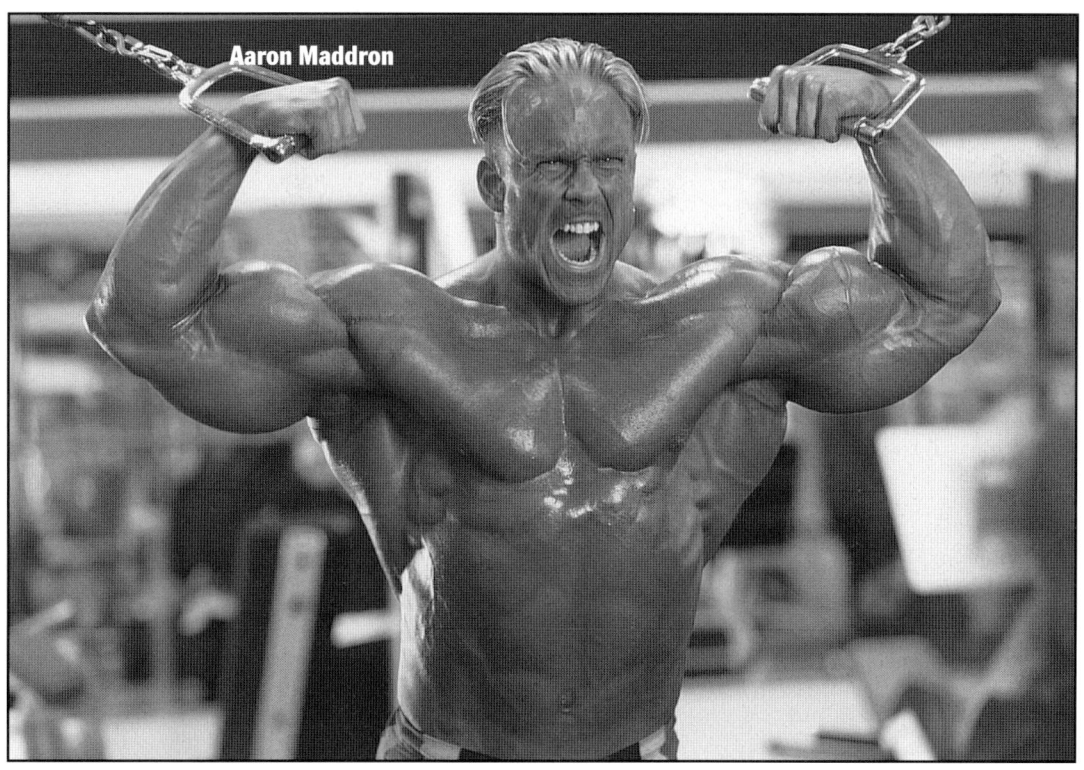
Aaron Maddron

CHAPTER SIX

each of the four steps as discussed in the past chapters you can start to shape the body you want. You do not need to buy some exotic machine to look great. Using the simple steps outlined in this program will do the trick.

In working with the four steps of the *Metabolic Magic* program it is important to allow your body enough time to get the job done. There are a lot of fad diets and programs that claim they can cause you to "lose 20 pounds in two weeks" or some other wild claim which are nothing more than that – wild claims. Rapid weight loss is extremely unhealthy. The body adapts gradually, and a gradual change is most likely to become permanent. With time and consistency the *Metabolic Magic* program will yield impressive results – results that you can keep if you make the four steps a habit pattern. Using tools such as weight training, cutting back on carbohydrate intake, increased duration cardio/aerobic training, and substituting fiber for fat all make a noticeable impact on the physique, and when added together as they are in the *Metabolic Magic* program, the combined impact over time can be quite significant and dramatic. Put each of the different steps into play, and get the most out of your physical potential.

You can shape a slender, slim and attractive physique if you use the right tools. The following chapter covers 20 hot tips and techniques to hype your metabolism, along with calorie and fat-burning activity charts.

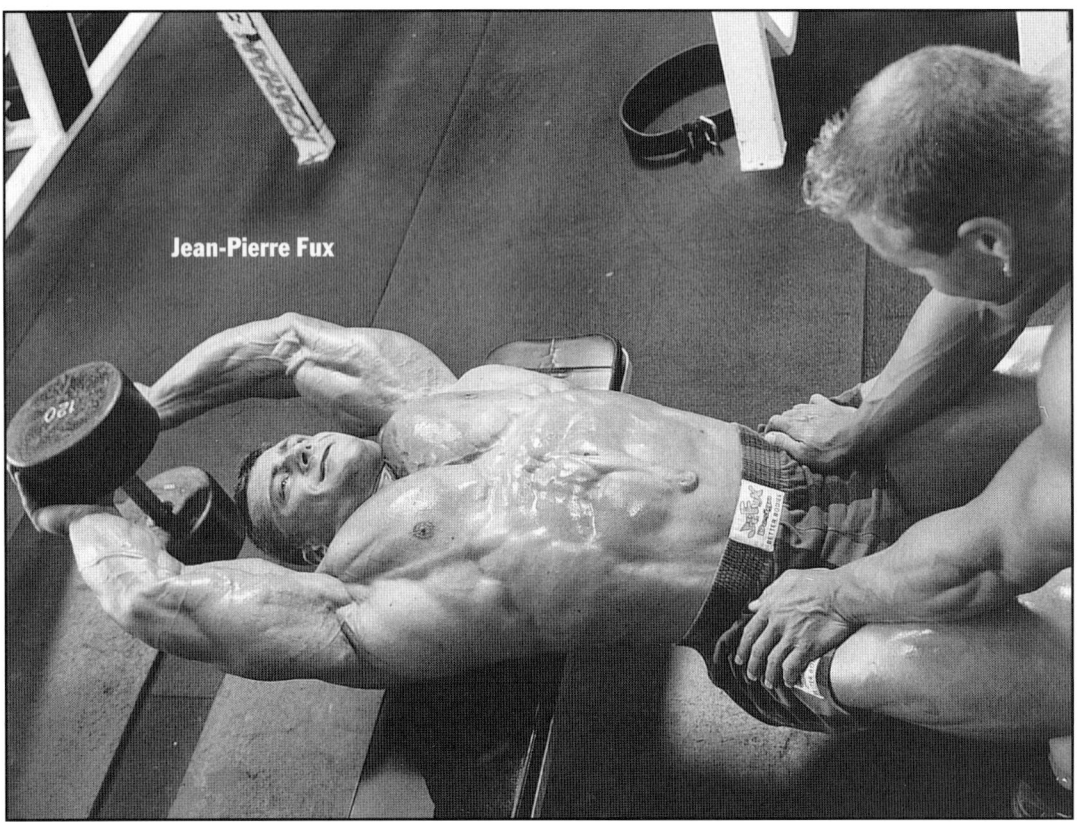

Jean-Pierre Fux

Metabolic Magic

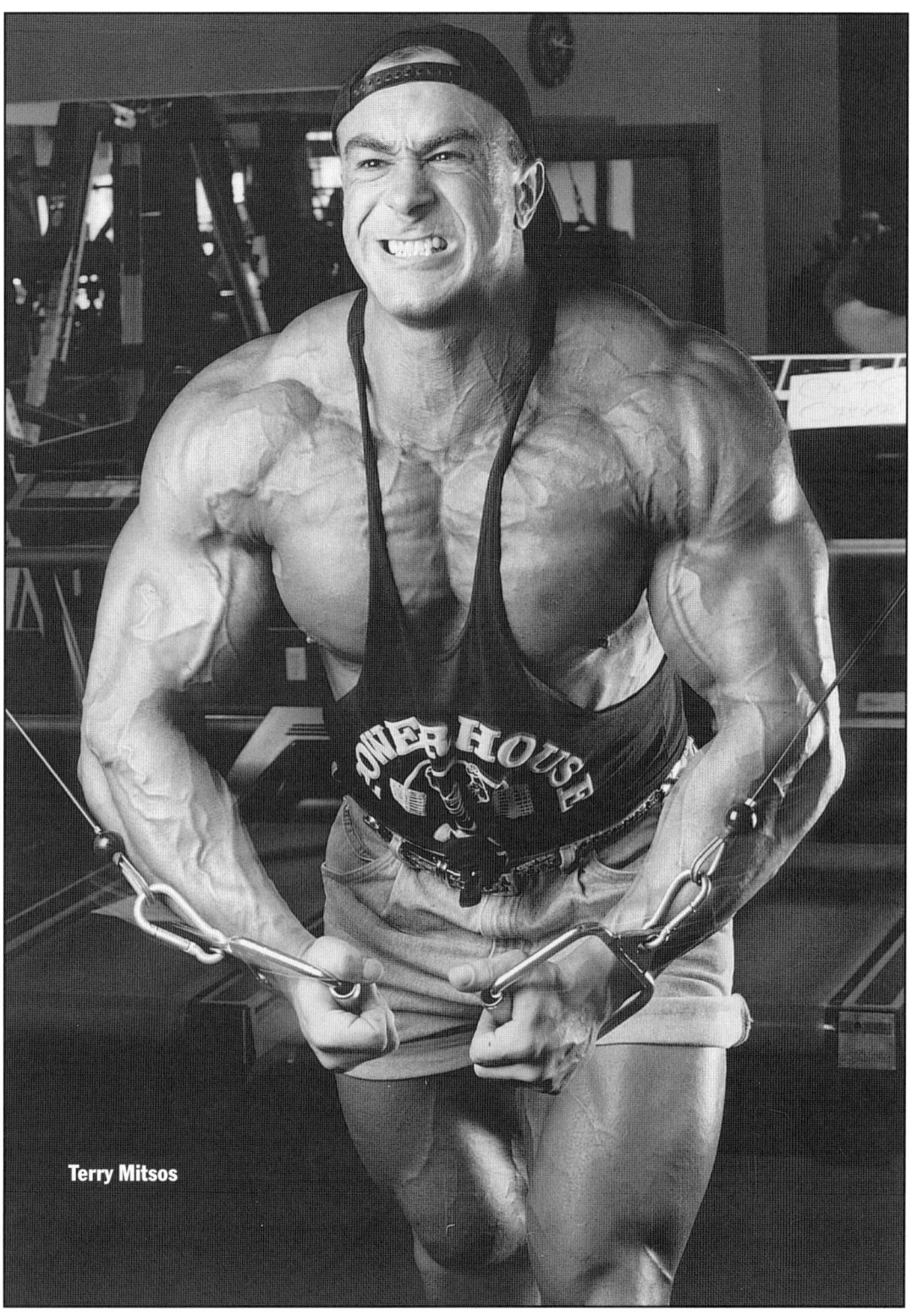

Terry Mitsos

CHAPTER SEVEN

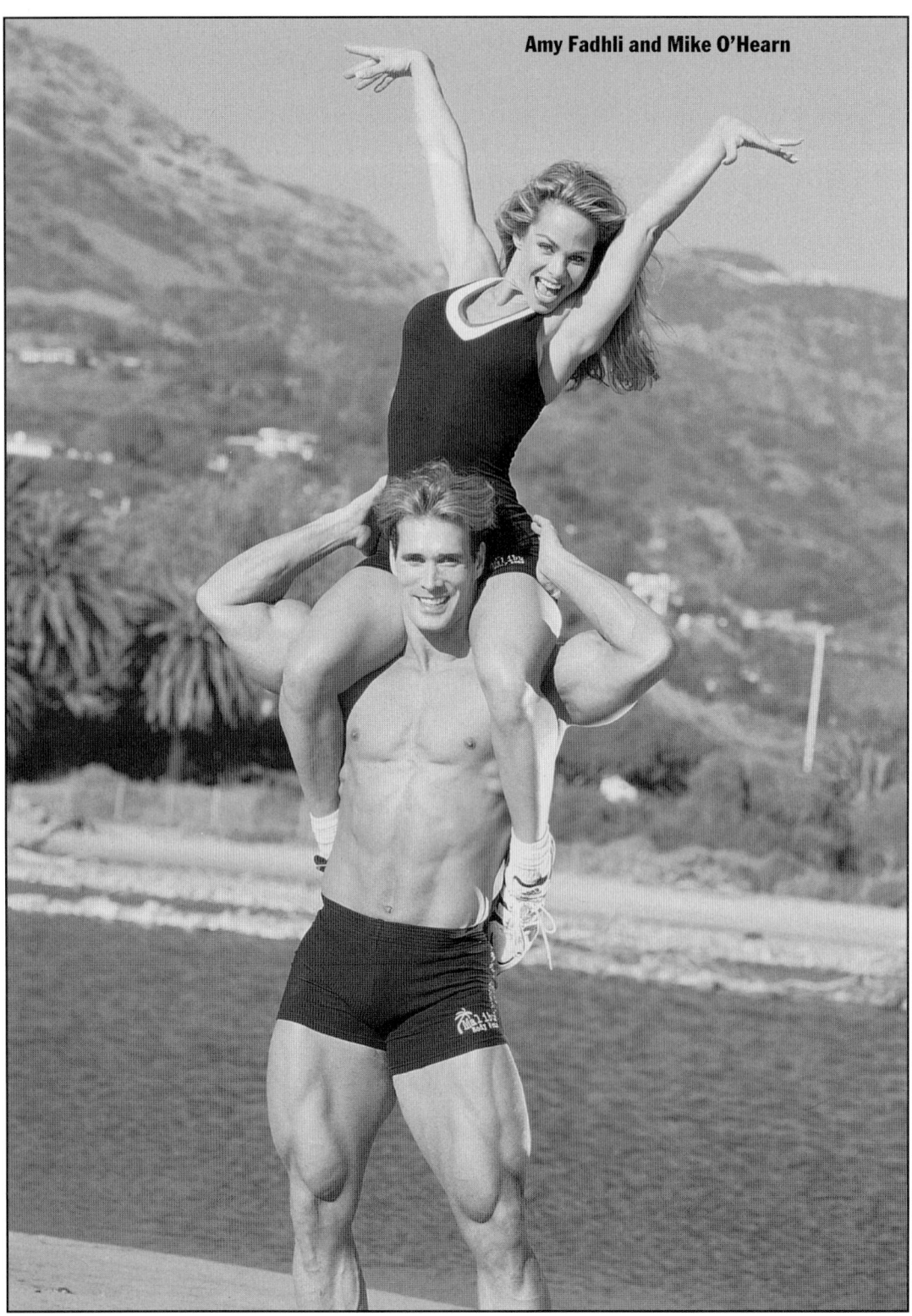

Amy Fadhli and Mike O'Hearn

20 Tips & Techniques to Hype Your Metabolism

"Hyping" your metabolism means gearing it up to a higher level. This is the most crucial element in burning off bodyfat – no other element comes close. The more "hyped" your metabolism is, the more fat you will use up throughout the day. Use these 20 hot tips and techniques which are part of the four steps to elevate your metabolism.

(1) Don't Sit – Move

Sitting around too much causes big problems for your physique. In addition to slowing down your metabolism, sitting is not good for the shape of your buns!

Sitting is a sedentary activity. Unfortunately, many people sit most of the time – at a computer terminal at work, in a car or bus on the way home, and then in front of the television in the evening. Sitting subtly and silently adds unwanted pounds to your body.

Instead of sitting as much as you normally do, consciously start standing and walking around more frequently. Take every opportunity to move your body instead of sitting down.

(2) Exercise Accumulation

Accumulate minutes of exercise activity throughout your day. Adults should accumulate 30 minutes or more of moderate-intensity physical activity on most, preferably all, days of the week. These recommendations

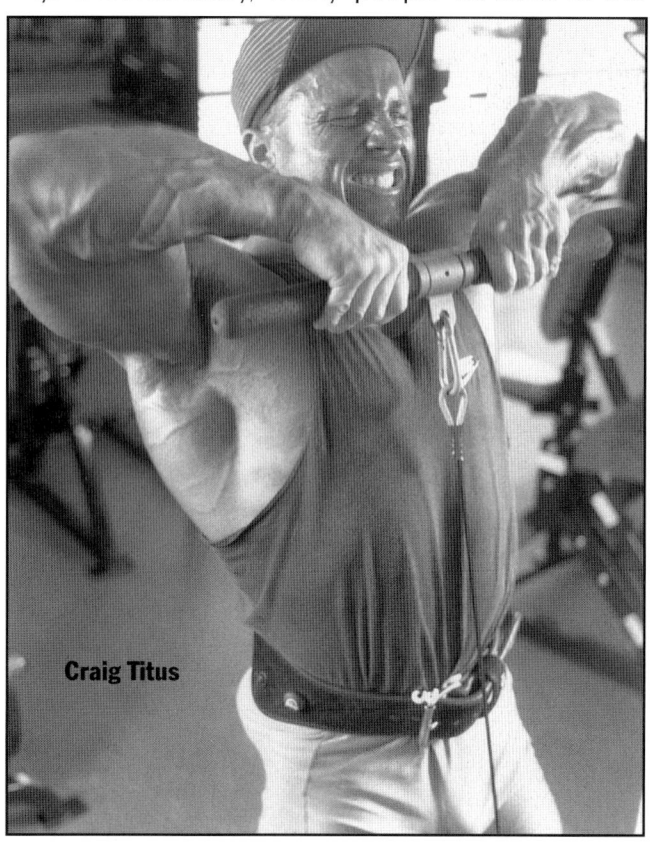

Craig Titus

37

CHAPTER SEVEN

emphasize the benefits of moderate-intensity exercise and activities that can be accumulated in short bouts throughout the day. Your activity does not have to come in one session alone or even in a formal exercise program to have an effect on your physique. Short and scattered periods of physical activity can benefit your body.

What does this accumulation of physical activity throughout the day do for you? It serves to increase your metabolic rate. And by doing it habitually you benefit your body on a continual basis. The more you are active during the day, the more time you build up of physical activity. This replaces the "sedentary slump" that most people succumb to. Throughout each day you are either active or not – you accumulate time of one or the other. There is no middle ground – so accumulate the right stuff – physical activity.

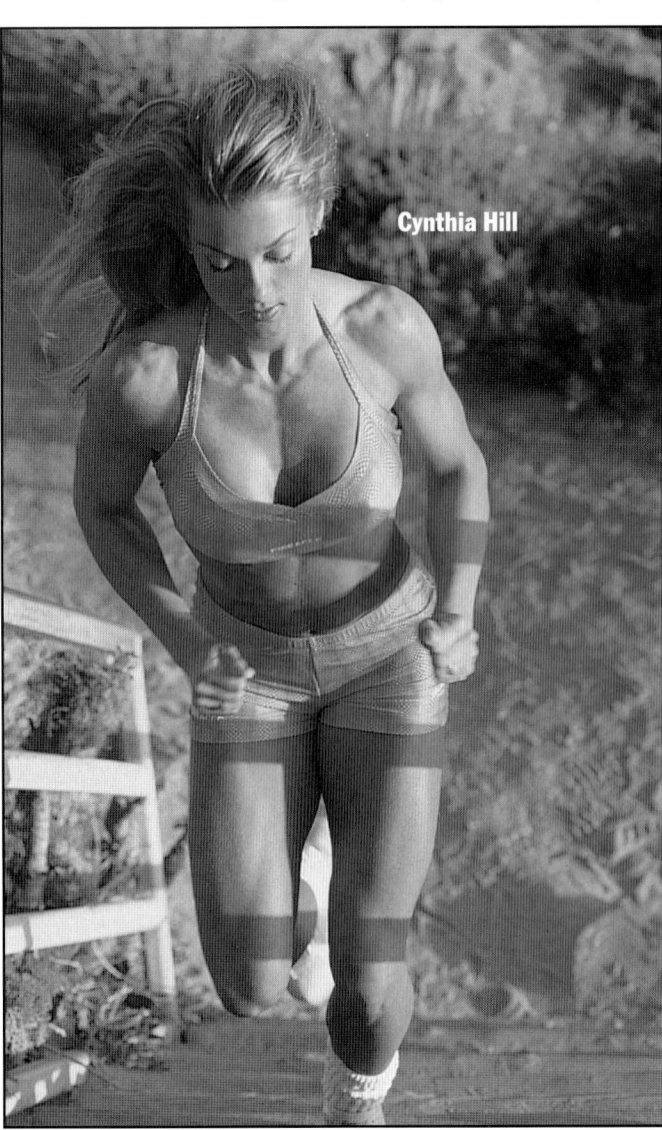

Cynthia Hill

(3) Stair Escape

What do you do if you are traveling and you have no access to a good gym? What if the motel you are staying at has no gym? Or what if it is closed for repairs or not open at the hour you need to use it? You may have to be up and gone by 7:00 A.M. and the gym does not open until 8:00 A.M. – what do you do? Motel/hotel stairs are better for more than just a fire escape – they can serve as an exercise escape as well. Hit the stairs for a good workout when you're on the road. Instead of sleeping in and letting your metabolism stay in low gear (as it often is on the road), get up and get going – up and down the stairs. Start your day with a stair workout and elevate your metabolism right away. You do not have to give up on your exercise just because you are on the road – plan to use the stair escape as an exercise escape.

Metabolic Magic

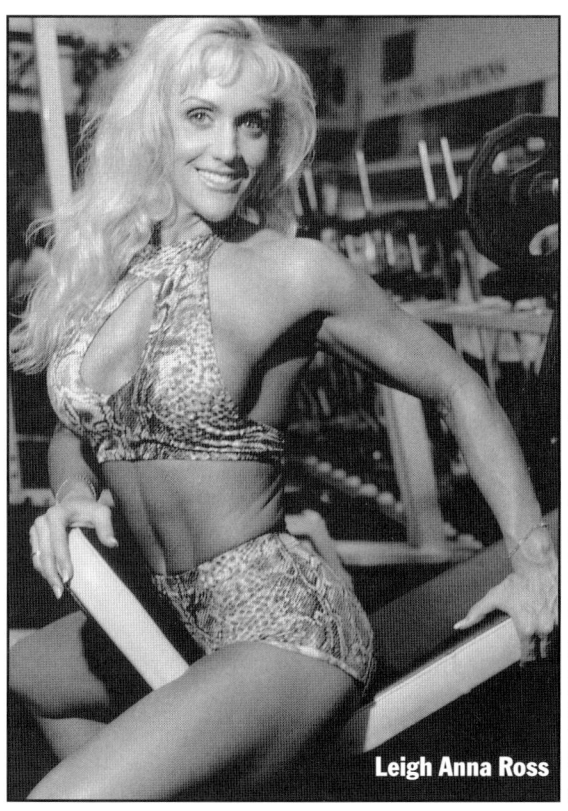

(4) Exercise in the P.M.

Would you like to burn more calories while you sleep? Exercise not only tones your muscles, it also fires up your physique's furnace – even hours after you have gone to bed. Research has shown performing an evening exercise routine that activates the major muscle groups can raise your metabolism by up to 10 percent higher than normal when you wake up the next day – 15 hours later.

One catch – not all exercise works equally well. The best booster of the metabolism is a strength training exercise like weight training. And hitting the major muscle groups is important – they really heat up your inner furnace. So get in some late night exercise to help your body burn those calories off as you sleep. Do more than dream at night – burn fat off as well.

Leigh Anna Ross

(5) Compound Concentration

Weight training is the premier manner in which to boost your metabolism, however, the way you utilize strength training will determine how much "metabolic hype" benefit you get from the exercise. Instead of performing specific exercises for the smaller muscle groups, aim at working the major muscle groups instead. The way to do this is with "compound" exercises. Compound exercises work more than one muscle group at a time. Bench presses, squats, pulldowns, clean-and-presses, etc. are a few examples of exercises that put more than one muscle group into play at once. When you attack the major muscle groups you really fire up your metabolism. And the concentration on compound exercises is very beneficial if you do not have a lot of time to spend on strength training. Simply focus on a few of the major muscle groups, boost your metabolism, and then get out of the gym.

(6) Sugar "Spike" Prevention

One of the more devastating occurrences that hits your metabolism is the sugar "spike". It is true that sugar does elevate your metabolism – but only for a very brief time. Soon thereafter you experience a corresponding plunge in your blood sugar. This "spike" wreaks havoc with your metabolism, slowing it down to a crawl. It is

CHAPTER SEVEN

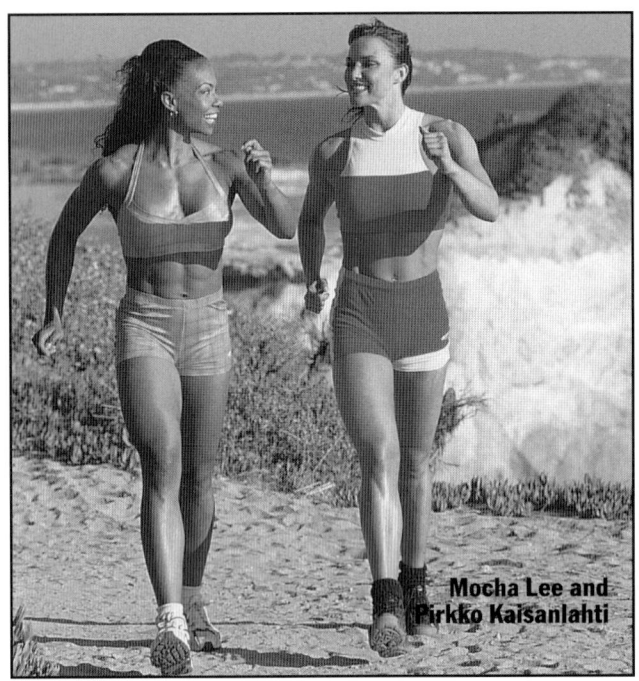

Mocha Lee and Pirkko Kaisanlahti

far better to keep your blood sugar at an even keel. It is easier to do this at home than on the road. Typically, when most people travel they tend to eat fast foods and other snacks that cause this nasty sugar "spike." Prepare "survival" kits for use on the road. These kits should contain fresh fruit, cut-up veggies, hard-boiled eggs, applesauce and low-fat pretzels. Instead of having to eat junk food or restaurant food, eat nutritiously.

Avoid the sugar "spike" that hits most often when you are on the go – prepare some nutritious foods ahead of time to give your body a steady flow of good fuel.

(7) Power Walking Power

Walking is a great exercise for burning off bodyfat. Although many people focus more on high-impact exercises such as running, walking fits the profile of a fat-burning activity better. Research from the Cooper Aerobics Center in Dallas pointed out that while you burn off calories faster doing more intense activities, you proportionally burn off more calories of fat when you walk. Remember more calories are burned from carbohydrate stores when you are using intense exercises, and more calories are burned from fat when you use moderate activities.

Walking is probably the top moderate-level activity that you can engage in – as long as you "power" walk. Power-walking provides just the right amount of stimulation to your body to burn fat instead of carbohydrates. One warning though, in order for power walking to be effective as a fat burning tool, you need to aim at a workout that is at least 30 minutes or longer.

(8) Metabolic Mix

Cardio/aerobic exercise trims off bodyfat during the workout, while weight training burns off bodyfat after the workout is over. Mix both together in your workout to maximize your metabolic boost. Mixing the two types of exercises helps you stay in top condition, and helps keep your metabolism "hyped". Mixing cardio/aerobics and weight training provides the ultimate tool for both muscle tone and metabolic elevation.

Metabolic Magic

(9) Water Workout

Weight training is a great way to fire up your metabolic furnace. However, it is not the only type of exercise that can bring about the much vaunted "post-workout" metabolic elevation. Water workouts can do the same thing. Swimming is more of a cardio/aerobic exercise, which means it does provide some fat-burning effects during the workout, but not much after the workout is over. However, swimming is not the only water exercise available. Aquatic fitness affords a way to simulate effects similar to that of weight training. Water provides 12 times the resistance of air and works against your movements in every direction. By performing exercises in the shallow end of the pool (such as standing leg kicks, etc.), you can stimulate the post-workout burn and also build up your muscle tone.

Water provides more than just an opportunity to get in the cardio/aerobic stimulation of swimming – it also gives you the chance to get in some aquatic fitness exercise and elevate your metabolism even more.

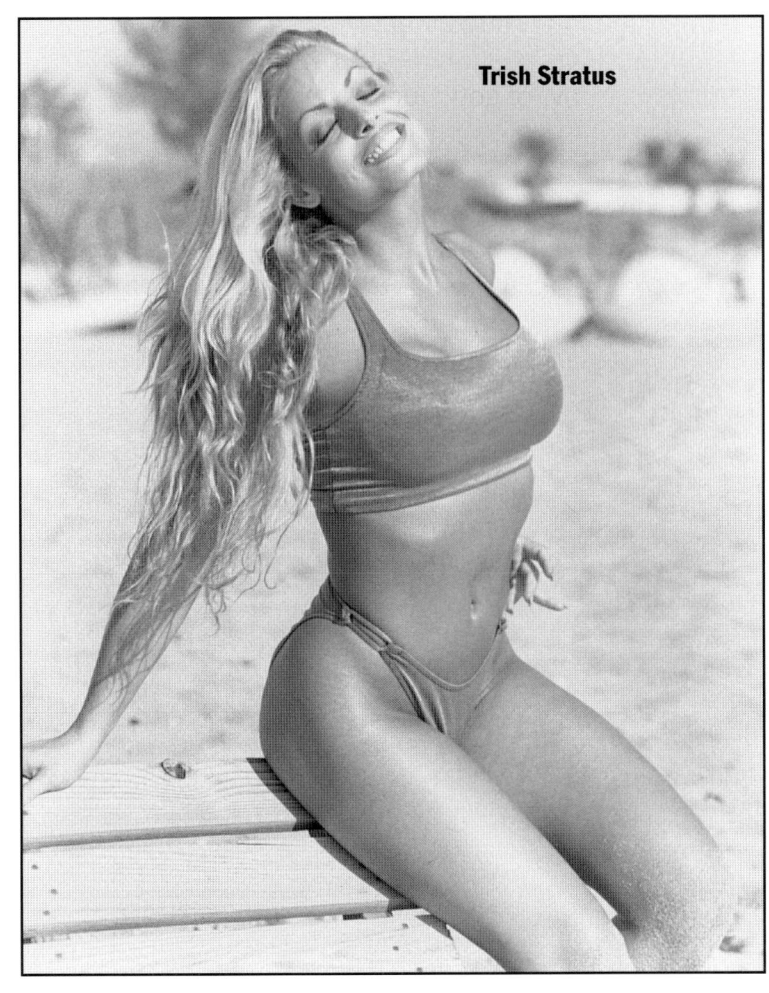

Trish Stratus

(10) Early Morning Exercise

As has been pointed out, working out later in the evening is great for elevating your metabolism. An early morning workout is also a good way to burn off unwanted bodyfat. Getting in an early morning workout starts your metabolism off in high gear for the day. Your body will turn to fat as a fuel source more readily in the morning than at other times because you have very little glycogen available. Make an early morning workout a habit for health and a "hyped" metabolism.

(11) Snack Attack

Most people love to snack. When it comes to snacking and the metabolism, often one of two mistakes are made. The majority of people spend time snacking on the wrong types of food – ice

CHAPTER SEVEN

cream (50 to 65 percent fat!), candy, pastries, etc. This provokes the undesirable sugar spike. Another common mistake is when people go on a diet they give up snacking altogether. This is not a good idea either. The best snacks to have are those high in fiber and complex carbohydrates. Eating these types of snacks can boost your metabolism in a positive, long-term manner.

(12) Jump-start Your Metabolism

In general, exercises that are of a moderate pace burn a higher percentage of bodyfat than do intensely active exercises. The one drawback with the moderate level exercise activities (such as power walking) is that they must be maintained for a fairly lengthy period. What do you do if you do not have 30-60 minutes available to work out? Some activity is far better than no activity. And if you do have a few minutes available, the exercise that packs the most into a short time period is jumping rope.

Jumping rope can get your metabolism elevated in a fairly short time period. You will not have the extended post-workout burn that weight training provides, but you will receive some metabolic uplift from jumping rope. And it provides several other benefits – health, coordination, stamina, etc., which all add up to enhance your appearance. So if you are caught in a time crunch – grab a rope and get in a fast workout.

(13) Frequent Meals

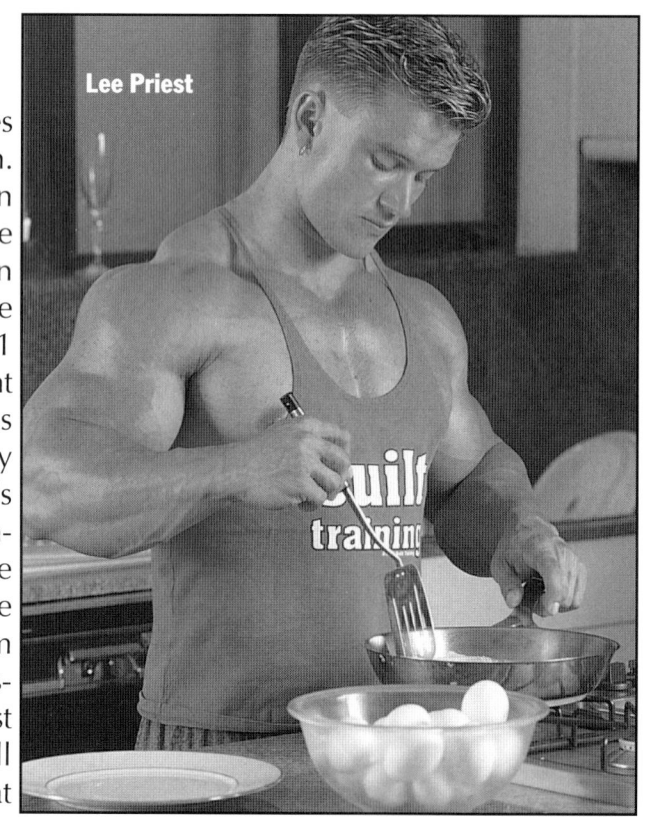

"Hyping" your metabolism usually takes discipline and effort to accomplish. However, there is one way that you can have some fun at it – through eating more frequently. When people diet, they often eat less frequently (according to the American Family Physician, about 21 percent of those who try to lose weight use this tactic). This is a big mistake. As you start to eat less frequently, your body slows its metabolic process to adjust. This is part of the reason (along with a sedentary lifestyle) that some people who are quite large eat very little yet remain quite large. By slowing down your metabolism (due to the decrease in the body processing your foods) you decrease the most powerful factor for fat loss – your overall metabolic rate. The meals that you eat should be smaller and nutritious. Eating more frequently won't help if you eat too many calories, particularly from fat and sugar sources. So eat more frequently, but make sure you are eating smaller meals that are composed of nutritious elements such as protein, fiber, and complex carbohydrates.

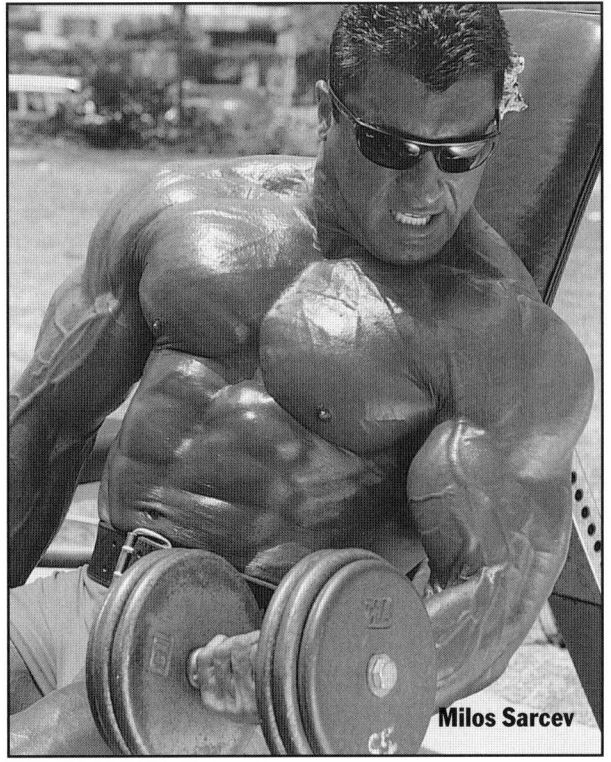

(14) Make Some Muscle

You can give your body a consistent boost in its metabolic rate by adding some muscle to your physique. Weight training builds muscle, and this muscle building process elevates your metabolism – often even into the next day. This gives you the great post-workout burn after every weight workout. However, you are not limited to just this effect. The more muscle you have, the higher your metabolism remains – lean muscle is more active even when at rest than fat. Many people go the the gym quite often yet don't seem to add any muscularity. The primary reason is that they do not increase the amount of weight that they use. Occasionally increasing the amount of weight that you use will stimulate your body to new levels of muscle tone and muscularity and this will in turn give you a consistently higher metabolic rate. So start the process as soon as possible by increasing the amount of weight that you use in your exercises.

Milos Sarcev

(15) Eat Early

Remember what Mom told you when you were growing up? Don't skip your breakfast! Pat Harper, a spokesperson for the American Dietetic Association, notes that if you eat most of your calories earlier in the day, you will actually stoke your internal fire to burn hotter. Another plus factor is that you have all day to burn the calories that you do eat off your physique. Research reveals that overweight people obtain 75 percent or more of their daily caloric intake in the evening, when the body is in a slow condition. This is a prime time for the body to store fat. Fight the problem by following the old adage – "breakfast like a king, lunch like a prince, and have dinner like a pauper." If you get more of your caloric intake earlier in the day and less later, you will give your metabolism a strong assist in staying "hyped" and hot.

CHAPTER SEVEN

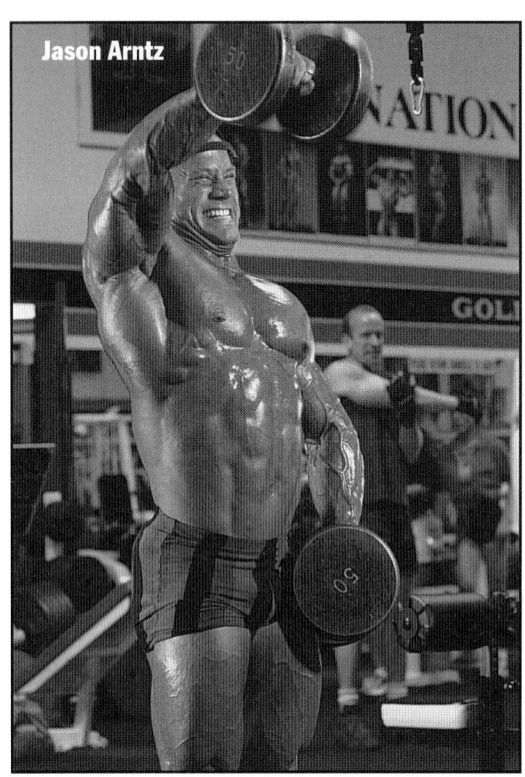

Jason Arntz

(16) Age Actively

An article in the *Journal of the American Medical Association* confirms what we have all long suspected – the total amount of time engaging in physical activity declines with age. This translates into a decreased metabolic rate as we age. However, the good news is that the decline in activity level (which in turn leads to an increase in bodyfat) is a variable factor. That means the problem can be addressed positively.

Many people plan on slowing down as they get older. If you want to look fantastic – with a trimmer physique than 99 percent of your peers, simply refuse to go along with that approach. Increase instead of decrease your activity levels. Doing so will keep your metabolism running at a higher clip.

(17) Metabolic Maintenance

Make "hyping" your metabolism a habitual practice. An article in the *New England Journal of Medicine* (August 7, 1997) noted that approximately two thirds of the people who lose weight will regain it within one year, and almost all persons will regain the weight within five years. The FDA has recently noted the same phenomenon. Don't become a statistic! Do not focus on only elevating your metabolism for the short term. Take a long-term view of the process. The *New England Journal of Medicine* pointed out that lifestyle changes in the form of increased exercise or decreased caloric intake made to lose weight will need to be continued indefinitely if the lower bodyweight is to be maintained. Gradually increase your exercise levels, decrease your caloric intake, and then stay at those levels. Aim at a long-term metabolic maintenance program if you want to look great and stay that way.

(18) Avoid Fad Drugs

Trimming down through "hyping" your metabolism is great – if you go about it in the right manner. There is a right way to fire up your metabolic rate, and there is a wrong way to go about the process. The right way is found throughout the pages of this book – using the information in a systematic and habitual approach. The wrong way is to take a short-cut approach. For many people, the short-cut involves some type of diet drug that is the fad of the month. Recent press attention has been given to the drugs phen-fen and Redux due to the health concerns related to intake of these substances. Drugs like these and others are only artificial props that will not give you long-term success, and will only serve to make you dependent upon them for your metabolic fix. What's worse, they endanger your health. Instead of using artificial means, use natural techniques to gain and maintain control of your metabolism.

(19) Turn up the Heat

You can add some zing to your foods and heat up your metabolism at the same time. In the book *Foods That Burn Fat*, it is noted that Dr. Jaya Henry of Oxford Polytechnic Institute of England found that the amount of hot mustard normally called for in a Mexican, Indian, or Oriental recipe dish (approximately a teaspoonful) temporarily speeds up the metabolism. The same is true of peppers. Dr. Henry found that peppers elevate the metabolic rate, giving what he terms the diet-induced thermic effect. Not much is needed to bring about this thermic effect. He points out that this tool for increasing the metabolism can be used every day. And unlike fad drugs, peppers and mustard are natural and totally safe.

Can you handle the heat? If you can, you can assist your metabolism in stepping up to a higher level. Consider adding more peppers and hot mustard to your meals on a consistent basis.

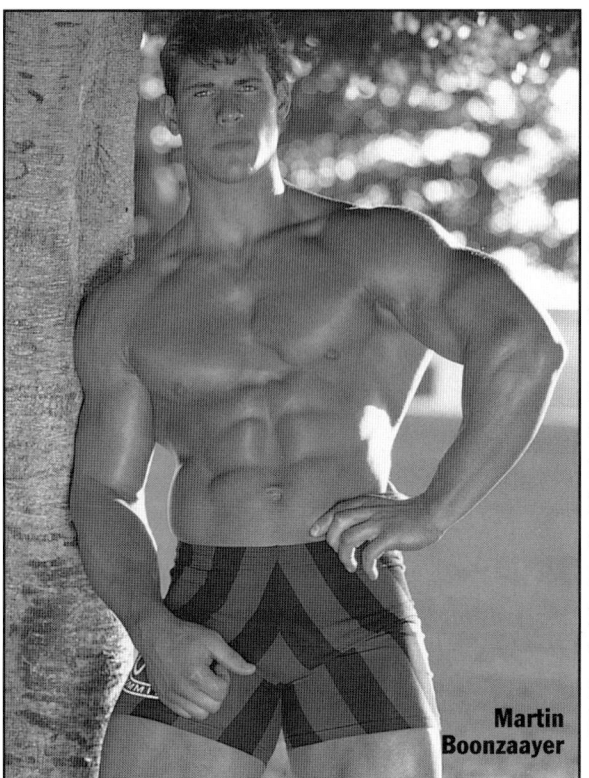

Martin Boonzaayer

(20) Metabolic Assist

You can assist your metabolic process by drinking more water on a daily basis. Water flushes fat and dangerous chemicals from the body's system, making weight loss easier. If you lack adequate water intake, you inhibit the metabolic process to some degree.

Most people do not now how much water they should be taking each day. The most common recommendations are for the intake of 1/2 to 1 gallon of water per day, with active people at the upper end of that range. And if you are working out frequently, especially in the heat, you will need even more water. Don't neglect this critical link in the metabolic process.

APPENDIX

Appendix A

Calorie Chart for Burning Off Bodyfat

	30 minutes	45 minutes	60 minutes
Backpacking	210 calories	315	420
Cycling (5 mph)	120 calories	180	240
Cycling (8-8.5 mph)	180 calories	270	360
Cycling (12 mph)	300 calories	450	600
Cycling (14 mph)	360 calories	540	720
Cycling (16 mph)	450 calories	675	900
Dancing	150 calories	225	300
Dancing (mod.-heavy)	240 calories	360	480
Jogging (5 mph)	300 calories	450	600
Light Calisthenics	120 calories	180	240
Light swimming	180 calories	270	360
Rollerblading	180 calories	270	360
Rollerblading (heavy)	330 calories	495	660
Running (5.5 mph)	330 calories	495	660
Running (6 mph)	390 calories	585	780
Running (7 mph)	450 calories	675	900
Running (8 mph)	480 calories	720	960
Running (9 mph)	510 calories	765	1020
Running (10 mph)	540 calories	810	1080
Stair climbing	180 calories	270	360
Stair climbing (mod.)	240 calories	360	480
Stair climbing (heavy)	300 calories	450	600
Walking (1-2 mph)	90 calories	135	180
Walking (2-3 mph)	120 calories	180	240
Walking (31/2-4 mph)	180 calories	270	360
Walking (4-4/2 mph)	210 calories	315	420
Walking (5 mph)	240 calories	360	480

Appendix B

Eating Right

One of the four simple steps outlined in *Metabolic Magic* is to reduce your carbohydrate intake. This should be done in a cycle – where you lower your carbohydrate intake for a period of time, then increase it again. This will help your metabolism burn off fat. In addition to the "low-carb cycle", you should otherwise maintain a diet that is healthy and nutritious, supplying your body with quality protein, fiber, carbohydrates and yes, even some fat (a small amount is necessary for the body's various functions) on a consistent basis. Your body needs these nutrients to function at an optimum level. Your body also needs the right amount of energy from food – not too much and not too little. Too much food energy and your body will be forced to store it as fat. Too little food energy and you will start to drag around and your metabolism will slow down.

Eat a good breakfast each morning, with some protein and complex carbohydrates as well as fresh fruit, if possible. Eating well at breakfast is good for your body. A few examples of a good breakfast include:

- **Three egg omelette with small potato, and juice**

Remove 2 yolks from the eggs. Mix the egg whites with the one yolk. Season eggs and potato to taste.

- **Turkey breakfast**

2-3 ounces of extra lean turkey breast, seasoned to taste
whole wheat toast, no butter (small amount of jam is okay)
skim milk.

- **Super cereal breakfast**

Oatmeal
skim milk
diced banana, raisins, and dates mixed into cereal with small amount of honey

These meals provide an idea for you to build your own. Have some quality protein from low-fat sources as well as complex carbohydrates and fiber.

Lunch

A healthy lunch contains a good balance of protein, carbohydrates and fats and enough calories to give you energy. 500-600 calories is ideal; 700 or more is too much. The perfect lunch for you could be:

- **Sandwich and a salad**

3 ounces of sliced turkey, whole grain bread, mustard and mayonnaise,
lettuce and tomato.
Side salad
Piece of fruit and a glass of skim milk
This meal provides 570 calories.

APPENDIX

• **Pita pocket sandwich**
pita bread
chicken chunks
light ranch dressing mixed with onions, cucumber, olives and lettuce
Enjoy with a glass of fruit or vegetable juice.

• **Burrito sandwich**
low-fat burrito shell
tuna
non-fat refried beans
tomato, cut into small pieces
light cheese
Eat with a small salad.

These ideas should get you started toward concocting your own nutritious low-fat meals for lunch.

Dinner

Dinner should be a smaller meal. Have a piece of meat (low fat) such as turkey, chicken, fish, etc., along with a salad and/or vegetable dish.

Snacks should follow the same pattern – a mixture of the essential nutrients in a low/calorie, low fat package. A good snack might include a cup of yogurt and a banana. Sunflower seeds (or peanuts) and a bagel. Super tip – mix some tuna into a cup of instant rice and beans for an outstanding snack.

Eating healthily will take some planning, but it will also pay off for you with a healthier body that has much more energy and less fat. And it will help you manage your metabolism much better, avoiding the nasty sugar spikes. Eat a well-balanced but low-calorie diet daily. And occasionally use a low-carb cycle to burn off a little extra bodyfat.

Contributing Photographers
Jim Amentler, Alex Ardenti, John A. Butler,
Paula Crane, Ralph DeHaan, Skip Faulkner,
Irvin Gelb, Robert Kennedy, Marconi,
Jason Mathas, Rick Schaff, Rob Sims, Art Zeller